Living with Lupus

Living *with* Lupus

THE COMPLETE GUIDE

Second Edition, Revised and Updated

Sheldon Paul Blau,
MD, FACP, FACR

Dodi Schultz

Da Capo

LIFE
LONG

A Member of the Perseus Books Group

Designed by Trish Wilkinson
Set in 11.5-point Goudy by the Perseus Books Group

Library of Congress Cataloging-in-Publication Data
Blau, Sheldon Paul, 1935–
    Living with lupus : the complete guide / Sheldon Paul Blau, Dodi Schultz.—2nd ed., rev. and updated.
        p. cm.
    Includes bibliographical references and index.
    ISBN 0-7382-0922-8 (pbk. : alk. paper)
    1. Systemic lupus erythematosus—Popular works. I. Schultz, Dodi. II. Title.
RC924.5.L85B555 2004
362.196'772—dc22

                                                                        2004012687

First Da Capo Press edition 2004

Published by Da Capo Press
A Member of the Perseus Books Group
http://www.dacapopress.com

Da Capo Press books are available at special discounts for bulk purchases in the U.S. by corporations, institutions, and other organizations. For more information, please contact the Special Markets Department at the Perseus Books Group, 11 Cambridge Center, Cambridge, MA 02142, or call (800) 255-1514 or (617) 252-5298, or e-mail special.markets@perseusbooks.com.

1 2 3 4 5 6 7 8 9—08 07 06 05 04

For Bette, Debra, Steven, and Ashley

Contents

CHAPTER

1

"Friendly Fire":
The Body Against Itself

It started when I was about thirty-eight or forty. I remember having really bad pains in my joints, just for a few days, with a rash on my cheeks—I'm pretty sure it was what they call the butterfly rash—and a little fever. I did go to the doctor, but the tests didn't show anything. And then it all went away—until it came back, about five years later.

❧

I was in my last year of high school. My hands hurt. It was weird, but all of a sudden my hands hurt. Not that much—but they kept hurting. My family doctor—that was in Pennsylvania— said it was mild rheumatoid arthritis. I didn't really think much more about it, just took some aspirin when it got really uncomfortable. It didn't really keep me from doing anything. And it never did get any worse.

Then, ten years later, I was married and I'd moved to just outside of Boston, and I got pregnant. There were a lot of complications, like thrombophlebitis and pulmonary emboli, and my obstetrician said, "I think you have a collagen disease." My baby was fine, and I felt pretty good after she was born, but my doctor warned me that I should never get pregnant again.

And I didn't. But then a few years later, I started feeling horribly tired all the time and getting these weird blisters on the roof of my mouth, and my obstetrician, who was now my gynecologist, said, "Why don't you see a rheumatologist?"

Looking back, I may have had a problem for years before it was diagnosed. I had a lot of things wrong from time to time, but I never connected them. The first thing I remember was that my feet started hurting. And there were changes in my menstrual patterns. My gynecologist said maybe it was early menopause—but I was only thirty-six!

Then everything went back to normal—until I started getting wrist pains, which I figured had something to do with working at the computer; my husband, Charlie, and I are partners, graphic designers. Then the foot pain came back, and then pain in my fingers. Then, my hair started to get thin, and I thought, well, I was forty by now, and my mother's hair has been thin for years, and I figured I was getting older. I decided that also accounted for the fact that the skin on my face was sort of dry and reddish. I was also tiring very easily.

I didn't put any of this together, and neither did my doctor. He just said that women my age often started getting aches and pains. About feeling tired, he said, "You're no spring chicken." And then it was November, a very busy time for us because clients are doing holiday promotions. And we had friends coming from out of town for Thanksgiving.

Now, I am not the kind of person who normally lets anyone help out in the kitchen—but the pain in my fingers and wrists was so bad, I really needed help picking up pots and pans, and I was grateful for it. And there was one other thing: I was having to go to the bathroom ridiculously often, and I finally realized why: My mouth was terribly dry all the time, and I'd gotten into the habit of keeping water, or juice, or a soft drink next to me all the time—next to my computer, and next to the bed at night—and I was drinking all these extra fluids, so of course I was having frequent urination.

I'd also developed terrible gum problems. On my next visit to the dentist, he found some ulcers in my mouth—which I hadn't even been aware of, because they didn't hurt. I told him about my talk with my internist and about some of my other problems. He said, "I think you may have lupus."

⤮

I had slept with exactly one person, and I was diagnosed as having syphilis in a routine screening test. In fact, I was treated for syphilis. I know now that was probably a false-positive test. Every once in a while, over the next ten years, I'd run low-grade fevers and feel kind of draggy, but my internist would say, "Oh, it's just a virus; don't worry about it."

Once, when I was around twenty-four or twenty-five—I was still living in L.A., where I grew up; that was before I moved to Oregon—one evening I was sitting in a movie theater, and my knees started to hurt. Later that night, I woke up and I couldn't move a single one of my joints; I had to call my parents to come across town and take me out of my apartment. I took a lot of aspirin, and it went away in about three days. Then it happened again a few days later. I'd been taking a sulfa drug for a bladder infection, and I finally realized I was allergic to it.

After that, I was perfectly fine, for about five years—and then all the other symptoms set in.

⤮

Actually, I'm pretty sure it started maybe twenty years ago, when I was in my early thirties. I was dead tired all the time, and running a fever nearly every day. My internist kept saying he suspected lupus, and he put me in the hospital for tests. At first, everything came back negative. One of the specialists suggested it was all in my mind, that I was concerned about aging. Aging? At thirty-one or thirty-two? Finally, although they never did come up with a diagnosis, they found enough abnormal results to prove it wasn't psychosomatic. That was a relief, but it would have been a lot easier on me to know what it was. I was sick—even the specialists finally agreed with that—but I came out with no diagnosis. My rheumatologist says now that it wasn't their fault, that the testing just wasn't as sophisticated then.

At first I had only one symptom. I was working at a landscaping firm—a job I really loved—and one day, I had this rash—just a rash, no fever or anything else, and I hadn't been bitten or stung. It wouldn't go away, and I finally saw a dermatologist. He said I'd probably developed an allergy to the sun, and if I could manage to do most of my work in the shade, a high-SPF sunscreen would probably do the trick. It didn't. I went to see a different dermatologist.

This guy took one look at me and said, "Do you have lupus?" I said, "What?" I'd never heard of lupus. Then he asked me if I had any joint pains. And, well, I did; I just hadn't thought much about it. He sent me to a rheumatologist. The rheumatologist did blood tests, and he concluded that yes, I had lupus.

So I went to my local library and looked it up. I took out an old medical book—very old, but it was the only one they had that mentioned lupus. It compared lupus to tuberculosis and said the life expectancy was three to seven years. I was very young, and I was very scared. Of course I know better now; it's been more inconvenient than life-threatening. But that book was very, very scary.

~&~

It must have been, let's see, eight years ago now. Age, mid-thirties. I'd just gotten my real-estate license a few months before that, and I was doing pretty well; this part of Florida was really growing. I had a bout of joint pain. My internist referred me to a rheumatologist, who did some tests, but they didn't seem to tell much, and the arthritis—that's what it was, but that just means inflammation, it doesn't tell you why—went away by itself.

I don't really know whether it had any connection with lupus. And I didn't have any other problems for maybe four and a half or five years. Then, in the winter, a couple of years ago, I had symptoms of Raynaud's; of course I didn't know what to call it, then, but my fingers would get cold and turn white. I was talking to a cousin who happens to be a doctor, and I mentioned it, and he said, you ought to see a rheumatologist.

So I went back to the same specialist I'd seen before, and that was lucky because she'd done tests—which didn't show anything at all—when I saw her about the arthritis. But now, it was really helpful that she had a record of those. She called them "baseline values," and she explained to me that there's a range of normal values for these things, and mine might be different from somebody else's, so it was great that she had a record of mine and not just some average figures. The new tests were positive, and they showed I have lupus. My doctor says that she isn't sure, but the arthritis a few years back could have been a kind of precursor of lupus, although she didn't feel I had lupus then.

Rash. Fever. Joint pains. Fatigue. Blood clots. Respiratory problems. Fatigue. Thinning hair. Falsely positive tests for infection. Fatigue. All are symptoms of lupus—or, possibly, not.

There are as many pictures, as many personal experiences, of lupus as there are people who have had it. Lupus is much like the elephant in an old folk tale. Having heard of elephants but never having seen one, a curious monarch directed his wisest advisors to go forth, find and examine the exotic beast, and return and describe it. Unfortunately, all of the sages were blind. Depending on what part of the elephant was encountered—leg, tusk, trunk, or tail—the animal was likened to a tree trunk, a spear, a serpent, or a rope.

The first experience with lupus is often recognized only in retrospect—seen at the time as something else or, often, simply an enigma. Only when lupus is finally suspected and diagnosed may it be clear that events that took place months or even years earlier were actually—or, at least, possibly—signs and symptoms of lupus.

Lupus—its full medical name is *systemic lupus erythematosus*—is a mysterious illness. Although various aspects of it were described as far back as the 1840s, and it was recognized as a systemic disease well over a century ago, the cause is still unknown and a cure still elusive.

Lupus is not transmissible from one individual to another; in no case has contagion even been suspected. In the vast majority of patients, it does not prove fatal. The illness might be viewed as, essentially, the opposite of AIDS, in which the immune system fails to fight off infectious agents—they cause what are often called "opportunistic infections"—that take advantage of the body's vulnerability.

Lupus is very different. In lupus, the body's defenses don't falter or flag. Rather, they become hyperactive, fiercely assaulting an individual's own tissues as if those tissues were offending intruders, foreign agents that must be destroyed or expelled. In the military, that sort of situation is known as "friendly fire"—an attack intended to destroy the enemy but inadvertently, tragically, through some mistaken transmission of signals, misdirected at our own forces.

The immune system is the body's military, its defense force—and in lupus and certain other conditions, that defense force is misdirecting its fire to attack its own kind, its own "side." In medical terms, it is as if one has developed immunity to oneself, and lupus is therefore classed as an *autoimmune* disease (the prefix "auto-" means "self");

indeed, it is considered the prototype, the prime example, of such diseases. Lupus is a battle of the body against itself.

There are quite a few autoimmune conditions. Some involve a single organ or system; diabetes mellitus, Graves' disease, and psoriasis affect respectively the pancreas, the thyroid gland, and the skin (sometimes the joints as well). In lupus, the targeted tissues may include the skin, joints, or vital organs, and evidence of lupus activity may range from a bothersome rash to critical kidney dysfunction. Lupus spans the gamut from a persistent nuisance to a threat to life—in different people, or in the same person at different times.

There is as yet neither prevention nor cure, nothing that will vanquish the disease. Although there may be periods of remission when little or no treatment is needed, lupus is chronic, a lifelong presence. But there are many effective ways of dealing with its manifestations, both its minor annoyances and its major complications.

It has been estimated that at least 1,400,000 to 2,000,000 Americans suffer from lupus. There is no official tally for lupus, such as those published by the Centers for Disease Control and Prevention for tuberculosis, AIDS, measles, and other diseases for which reporting to public health authorities is mandated. The cited estimates of lupus prevalence are undoubtedly low. They are based on a survey commissioned by the Lupus Foundation of America, with results reported in 1994, and they reflect diagnosed cases only. The true total is doubtless considerably higher.

Prior to that survey, published estimates—generally based on physician surveys—were even lower. One reason for the probable underestimates in such surveys was the practice of not counting those patients whose symptoms were limited to the skin. Until recently, it was held that such cases constituted a completely distinct disease, known as "discoid lupus," named for the characteristic skin lesions, which are raised and roughly disk-shaped. It's now recognized that discoid lupus is simply a part of the lupus spectrum.

Another reason for low prevalence estimates is that many cases never enter the database. Many instances of the disease, due to the nature of its manifestations, may simply escape medical attention entirely.

In general, estimates of noncontagious, nonreportable disease prevalence rely on some sort of official records such as hospital discharge logs, emergency-room visits, and reasons noted for school absences. It is thus possible to estimate numbers of heart attacks, broken legs, and children suffering from severe asthma, for example, with reasonable accuracy.

Most people with lupus, most of the time, continue to go about their daily lives. They're predominantly adults and, like most, often report to their jobs even when they're not feeling quite up to par; or they may avail themselves of allotted "sick days" or "personal leave days," without reporting the reason. They may be self-employed. They may be college students or homemakers and therefore not counted in the "work force." Unless their symptoms become life-threatening, they don't appear in emergency rooms, and thus, they don't become statistics.

Through the 1980s or so, many of the generally accepted estimates of lupus prevalence relied chiefly on hospitalization data. Research conducted in the early 1990s, however, revealed that fewer than half of lupus patients are likely to be hospitalized within any ten-year period (in the experience of many physicians, the proportion is significantly lower, perhaps 10 or 15 percent). In short, most lupus patients simply aren't enumerated anywhere. Thus, an assumption that hospitalized lupus patients represent a high proportion of the total number of lupus patients is likely to lead to gross underestimates of that total.

Although lupus has been diagnosed in both small children and senior citizens, the concentration of cases (at the time of diagnosis) occurs during the period from the teen years through the forties, with a mean onset age of twenty-nine or thirty. During these years of highest incidence, the female-to-male ratio is at least nine to one (after the mid-fifties, it drops to around two to one). No one is sure why this sex difference exists.

Lupus, as every lupus patient knows, is a frustrating experience. Your physician cannot explain its cause, predict its course, or promise a cure. This bafflement, this inability of medicine to clarify the nature and outcome of lupus has led, as many medical mysteries do, to speculation, to theories, to a continuing search for solutions. It has also led, at times, to the spreading of outrageous misinformation.

Until the 1970s, lupus was little known to the public or even to writers of popular home health guides, and many books published before that time dismissed lupus as "rare," or as "a disease of the skin." Still older books, possibly confusing what we now call lupus with other diseases, characterized it as invariably deadly, frightening a great many recently diagnosed patients who encountered these very old works in libraries. And there have been many other misunderstandings over the years, with confused journalists describing lupus as everything from a familial curse to a sexually transmitted scourge.

It's true that a few well-known Americans have died of complications of lupus. The best-known was probably the gifted novelist and short-story writer Flannery O'Connor, who died in 1964. More recently, in 1997, the veteran broadcast journalist Charles Kuralt succumbed to the disease, as did actor John Wayne's eldest son, Michael, who, according to news reports, died of lupus-related heart failure in 2003 at the age of sixty-eight.

Lupus is in fact *not* often fatal. Many examinations of survival rates in lupus patients have been published over the years—and a significant difference has emerged over those years. A summary published in 1955 showed a five-year survival rate of only 50 percent. By the 1990s, both the five- and ten-year survival rates were in the mid-90 percent range, and the twenty-year figure was over 85 percent. As one might expect, the tremendous jump in these survival rates is rather deceptive, for reasons similar to the distortions in the early prevalence estimates.

Treatment of lupus has indeed advanced tremendously in the past half-century, and the outlook for the patient is far rosier now than it was earlier. But diagnosis has also come a long way. The 1955 survival rate of only 50 percent was doubtless based on only a fraction of those who actually had lupus—that is, only those patients who were hospitalized—and those certainly represented the most serious and complicated cases. Thus, since the total number of people with lupus was significantly underestimated, published mortality rates—calculated as a proportion of that presumed total—appeared much higher than they actually were.

Even today, many cases of lupus escape diagnosis, so the most recently published survival rates are probably on the low side, as well. That is, since the true total is doubtless higher than estimated on the basis of surveys, those who die of the disease likely constitute an even smaller proportion of all lupus patients than is estimated.

Today, although lupus can be neither prevented nor cured, there is much that *can* be done, by both patient and physician. If a crisis does occur, your physician can now summon sophisticated diagnostic and therapeutic technology to your aid, and the efficacy of that technology is steadily increasing. Chances are, however, such a crisis will not occur; as we've said, only a small minority of lupus patients are ever sick enough to require hospitalization.

The vast majority of those with lupus never face a major crisis; they simply cope, on a day-to-day basis, with what may seem at times to be a succession of *minor* crises. Some of that coping can be aided by your physician, who can prescribe and suggest ways to ease discomfort and to deal with the disease's vexingly unforeseeable course. Some is best done by you.

There is now a greater understanding of lupus and its physical and emotional impact. There is new thinking, and there are new therapies—not only medical treatment but additional steps a patient can successfully take to relieve and to prevent problems.

This book shares that information, along with the latest from the medical research front. We hope that if you have lupus, or someone you care about has lupus, you'll gain new insight into, and appreciation of, *living* with lupus.

A NOTE ON NAMES

Some readers may be puzzled by the name of the disease. Why is it called "lupus"? Before we go on to explore the various facets of living with lupus in the twenty-first century, a brief explanation, as well as comment on some persistent confusion, is in order.

Lupus is the Latin word for "wolf." It was first used medically in the mid-nineteenth century to denote a completely different condition, a "malignant ulceration often destroying the nose, face, &c" (the definition in the first US medical dictionary).[1] Someone probably thought the damage caused by the disease resembled the result of an attack by a ravenous wolf.

The full medical term for that disease, which is totally unrelated to the condition now called lupus, was lupus vulgaris (the latter Latin word simply means "common" or "ordinary"). A variant form of the disease, characterized by very large, reddish nodules, was labeled lupus tumidus or lupus hypertrophicus. All of those terms are now obsolete, and the modern name for the disease is cutaneous (affecting the skin) tuberculosis. This form of TB results in extensive ulceration and tissue destruction and affects the face, especially around the nose and cheeks and sometimes the chin, more often than other sites. The cause is the same bacterium that typically targets the lungs but may occasionally attack other parts of the body. In the 1850s, its infectious cause was unknown; the tuberculosis bacillus, *Mycobacterium tuberculosis*, wasn't identified until 1882.

Some years earlier, in the 1840s, the Viennese physician Ferdinand von Hebra had described a distinctive rash—"mainly on the face, on the cheeks and nose in a distribution not dissimilar to a butterfly." This is, of course, the now-famous "butterfly rash," which is probably the best-known characteristic of lupus, although it appears in only about half of cases. Dr. Hebra's description was the first in the medical literature of the condition we now know as lupus.

Clearly, this was not the destructive affliction then known as lupus vulgaris, although it seemed to affect the same area. Since it was a different condition, a different name was needed. In 1851, the French dermatologist Pierre Cazenave combined the Latin word already in use with a new Greek-rooted French one and introduced the term lupus erythemateux, "lupus characterized by redness." The second word was soon Latinized to erythematosus. Later, after it had been conclusively demonstrated that the condition affects various parts of the body, "disseminated" was added up front. Still later, that was changed to "systemic," and the full medical term became systemic lupus erythematosus, or SLE. Now, patients and physicians alike refer to the disease simply as "lupus."

NOTES

1. C. H. Cleaveland, M.D., *Pronouncing Medical Lexicon, Containing the Correct Pronunciation and Definition of Most of the Terms Used by Speakers and Writers of Medicine and the Collateral Sciences* (Cincinnati: Longley Brothers), 1857.

2

The Difficult Diagnosis

How does a physician arrive at the conclusion that a patient is suffering from lupus? The diagnosis isn't an easy one, especially for a physician who is inexperienced. Many people visit three, four, or more doctors before lupus is either confirmed or eliminated from consideration.

The diagnosis should be made by a specialist, a rheumatologist, for a number of reasons, including familiarity with the spectrum of the disease (and related ills with which it can be easily confused) and awareness of the latest scientific information in the field. A primary-care physician, a general internist or family physician, or another physician or dentist who suspects the possibility of lupus will generally refer the patient to such a specialist. Unfortunately, some practitioners fail to suspect that possibility.

> The first doctor I saw said I was just tired and depressed; I don't know if he thought the fatigue caused the depression or vice versa, but he was sure that I wasn't sick. It was four more doctors and three more years before I found out what I actually had.

In a patient survey conducted by the American Autoimmune Related Diseases Association and reported in 2002, the majority of those with serious autoimmune diseases were found to have had significant problems in arriving at a diagnosis. Many were told that their symptoms were merely "in their heads" or that they were simply suffering from "stress." No fewer than 45 percent had in fact been labeled hypochondriacs.

Certainly, if you suspect that you may have lupus or another similar condition, your concerns should not be dismissed—nor should you accept such a dismissal. You should persist and insist on thorough investigation by a qualified specialist. That specialist is a *rheumatologist*; rheumatology is a subspecialty of internal medicine.

Arriving at a diagnosis, even for the experienced rheumatologist, is still not a simple matter. A strep infection can be identified by the presence of bacteria in a test-tube culture; the diagnosis of diabetes can be made by measuring insulin responses. No such simple test exists for lupus. Rather, the physician will arrive at a conclusion—and be aware that it may be tentative—based on the following:

- **The patient's complaints.** Lupus may begin with any one or more of a vast spectrum of symptoms, including—but not limited to—fever, fatigue, stomach upset, hair loss, rashes, and assorted aches and pains. Of course, all of these can be symptoms of many other conditions as well: allergic reactions, infections, and hormonal imbalances, to name just a few. There is, in particular, a great potential for overlap and confusion with other conditions in the "family" of which lupus is a part, generally known as the *connective-tissue diseases*—prominently, rheumatoid arthritis, progressive systemic sclerosis (scleroderma), myositis, and dermatomyositis.

  Sorting out the possibilities, a process known in medicine as *differential diagnosis,* is the challenge the physician faces. Depending on the individual patient's signs and symptoms, the physician may need to perform a number of tests and other procedures to eliminate other diseases and disorders.

  Of course, an experienced physician's first concern is the possibility of an acute condition that requires immediate action, whether or not that condition is associated with lupus. So the first considerations will be such possibilities—malignancies, serious infections, dysfunctions of major organs. Once they have been deemed unlikely, and lupus or another connective-tissue disease is strongly suspected, further exploration will be in order.

- **Established diagnostic criteria.** For each of the connective-tissue disorders, a set of descriptive guidelines have been developed by the Diagnostic and Therapeutic Criteria Committee of the American College of Rheumatology (ACR)—not a "college" in the generally understood sense but the professional organization of those physicians specializing in the treatment of the various forms of arthritis as well as other disorders involving autoimmune reactions.

  Patients (and physicians, too) must understand that these criteria do *not* represent a "test" that must be passed before someone can be said to have lupus. Rather, they serve a dual purpose. Primarily, they provide commonality of language; if physicians are to talk about treatment, explore causes, conduct trials of medications, and so forth, they must agree on a description of the disease they're discussing. Second, they provide confirmatory support for the practicing physician, a kind of diagnostic yardstick.

- **"Unofficial" factors.** The physician's own knowledge and experience frequently suggest other significant factors, beyond the "official" criteria.

  The ACR criteria are based on surveys of leading rheumatologists in the United States and Canada. They were established in the early 1980s, replacing tentative criteria proposed a decade earlier, and were revised in the late 1990s. The list may be further revised in the future, as more reliable, sensitive, and, especially, more specific diagnostic tests are developed and reaffirmed.

Before we go on to describe both the ACR criteria and other diagnostic determinants, a brief explanation is needed of two of the terms above, which have been used here in a particular medical sense.

SENSITIVITY AND SPECIFICITY

Diagnostic testing relies on two concepts, *sensitivity* and *specificity*. The first term refers to whether a test is likely to miss many cases of the disease or disorder for which the patient is being tested. The second refers to whether the test is helpful in narrowing the diagnosis to the condition being tested for.

Let's say, for example, that 95 percent of those with a condition we'll call "Dreaded Disease" have factor X in their blood. An accurate test for factor X would be positive in nineteen out of twenty people with Dreaded Disease, "missing" only one in twenty cases; it would be highly sensitive and thus useful for screening large populations.

If factor X is also found in 40 percent of perfectly healthy people, however, or in 40 percent of those with an entirely different disease, a positive result would not really be very helpful in pinpointing true cases of Dreaded Disease. Thus, a test for factor X would be low in specificity and thus not very useful for an individual patient's diagnosis.

Or, let's say there's another clue, called factor Y, that is found in 50 percent of those with Dreaded Disease but in only 1 percent of people who don't have the disease. An accurate test for factor Y could not be called sensitive, since in random screening it would miss half the cases of the disease—all those cases occurring in people with the disease but without factor Y. On the other hand, it would be far more specific than the test for factor X: A positive test for factor Y would mean 99-to-1 odds that the patient has Dreaded Disease.

Ideally, an accurate diagnostic test for a particular disease would be based on a characteristic found in *all* people with the disease and in *no one* without it. It would be 100 percent sensitive and 100 percent specific: A negative test would be guaranteed assurance that the patient doesn't have the disease (since the test wouldn't miss any cases), and a positive test would tell the physician the patient definitely has the disease (and not some other disease, or no disease at all). No such test yet exists for lupus, for the simple reason that it would rely on testing for a factor both unique to lupus and present in all cases of the disease. No such factor has yet been found.

Therefore, a combination of scientific knowledge, experience, and judgment are needed for diagnosis.

THE ACR DIAGNOSTIC CRITERIA

Of the American College of Rheumatology's current criteria for lupus, four are considered necessary to confirm the diagnosis without question, but the four needn't be present simultaneously. Some of the criteria are symptoms experienced by the patient or observable by both patient and physician; others must be determined by blood tests or other procedures.

Remember that this list, first drawn up more than three decades ago and already twice revised, is subject to future revision. Remember, too, that the criteria have been established chiefly to provide a common-ground basis for discussing the disease, not as a "test" the patient must pass. Many patients who unquestionably have lupus—perhaps half of all those who do—will *never* fully meet the ACR research-oriented criteria.

- **Butterfly rash.** A reddish eruption across the bridge of the nose and winging out over the cheekbones, in a sort of butterfly configuration. As noted in Chapter 1, it was this characteristic rash that gave the disease its name. It is often cited as a classic symptom of lupus—probably more due to its picturesque name than its prevalence. The rash isn't necessarily itchy or particularly painful, although it may burn slightly on exposure to the sun; it usually goes away and leaves no residual marking.

> I was the one who suspected I had lupus, after I'd read about it. But when I went to see the doctor who took care of me then and said, "Do you think maybe I might have lupus?" he said, "You can't possibly have lupus. You don't have the butterfly rash, and all those with lupus have the rash."

Some physicians are clearly unacquainted with the relatively low incidence of the butterfly rash, especially as an early symptom of lupus. It's an initial symptom in fewer than one in twenty cases of lupus, and only 40 to 60 percent of lupus patients (reported surveys have varied) will *ever* have it.

- **Discoid lesions.** Reddish, raised patches, anywhere on the body, sometimes referred to as discoid lupus erythematosus (DLE), which used to be classified as a disease distinct from systemic lupus erythematosus (SLE). DLE is now considered to be a part of the lupus spectrum, even if it is the only firm evidence of the disease. The lesions are roughly disk-shaped, thick, and scaly, and they may leave scars after healing.

  This kind of skin lesion occurs in about 15 percent of lupus patients, and in only 5 to 10 percent of those who have it does the disease affect other parts of the body. Some observers believe that one of the reasons for past low estimates of lupus prevalence is that DLE cases had, by and large, been omitted.

- **Photosensitivity of the skin,** with a rash specifically following exposure to sunlight or, often, fluorescent lights. This is often the very first symptom. Although only about one-third of those with lupus are light-sensitive, the reaction should suggest the possibility of lupus to any physician, especially if exposure correlates not only with skin manifestations but with other symptoms as well.

- **Ulcerative sores,** often (but not necessarily) painless, in the mouth or throat, and occasionally in the vagina. Sometimes, the patient is unaware of the oral lesions, and it's a dentist who notes them, perhaps during a routine checkup. When they first arise, they may be blister-like in appearance. About one in eight lupus patients has such sores at some time.

- **Arthritis**—joint inflammation, characterized by pain on motion, stiffness, tenderness, and swelling—in two or more peripheral joints. (Peripheral joints are those of the hands, arms, feet, and legs.) Joint aches, which are much like those of rheumatoid arthritis, are among the first symptoms in three of four cases of lupus, and at least 90 percent of patients will have arthralgia (joint pain) or arthritis sooner or later; its severity may vary considerably. The earliest arthritis symptom (in both lupus and rheumatoid arthritis) is usually morning stiffness of the fingers and wrists.

Joint pains, despite their prevalence in lupus patients, constitute a very nonspecific symptom. Not only are joint aches preeminent symptoms of such related ills as rheumatoid arthritis and osteoarthritis; they also can be—and often are—due to injury or to simple physical stress. They can also accompany a variety of acute infections, including rubella, Lyme disease, and ordinary influenza. In a 2001 survey of adults in the United States, fully one-third of all respondents—a proportion representing nearly 70 million people—reported that they'd suffered from joint pain.

Rheumatoid arthritis, the chief feature of which is joint pain and inflammation, is the disease most commonly confused with lupus when the patient's chief complaint focuses on joint discomfort. Some of the laboratory tests, however, may be helpful in distinguishing between them, as may the particular joints involved and how they are affected; X rays can sometimes help to reveal crucial differences. In general, in lupus, as contrasted with rheumatoid arthritis, any actual deformities in the joints are almost always confined to the hands and wrists, and erosion of the bone does not occur. At times, symptomatic confusion and inconclusive laboratory tests will result in a tentative diagnosis of "rhupus"—which simply means that it's not yet possible to affix a definite label.

- **Chest/heart problems.** Evidence of either pleurisy (pleuritis; inflammation of the pleura, the membrane lining the chest cavity) or pericarditis (inflammation of the pericardium, the outer membrane surrounding the heart). The patient has usually complained of chest pain, and the physician will order a chest X ray and electrocardiogram (ECG) to investigate.

Various studies have shown that one-third to approximately 45 percent of those with lupus have pleurisy at one time or another, though not necessarily initially, and about 25 percent will experience pericarditis.

- **Renal (kidney) disorder.** Kidney problems may be suggested by persistent proteinuria, the presence of certain proteins in the urine, or by discovery in the urine of elements known as cellular casts, which are fragments of red cells. Urinalysis is a standard part of the differential diagnosis, since it can also reveal additional conditions such as diabetes and urinary tract infections.

    Perhaps half of all lupus patients will have some degree of kidney involvement at some time. Reported figures have ranged, in various studies, from 40 to 75 percent, but most have been in the lower part of that range.

- **Signs of neurologic disorder.** Seizures and/or psychosis, occurring without any explanation. There are many other causes, including toxic drugs, injury, and metabolic derangement; infection is also a possible cause of sudden seizures. If there are such symptoms, diagnosis may require an electroencephalogram (EEG) and a lumbar puncture ("spinal tap") to obtain a sample of the cerebrospinal fluid that bathes the brain and flows down through the spinal canal, as well as other investigative procedures. Such disorders affect a small but significant proportion of those with lupus, perhaps 15 percent.

- **Hematologic (blood) abnormalities.** These may include hemolytic anemia (caused by too-rapid destruction of red blood cells), leukopenia (a deficit in white cells), or thrombocytopenia (a deficit in thrombocytes or platelets, the clotting cells); a symptom of the last may be "bruises" in the absence of injury, caused by spontaneous bleeding of small vessels in the skin, or the persistent refusal of an injury to heal properly. A complete blood count (CBC) is, of course, a basic diagnostic procedure. Just about all lupus patients will have some hematologic departure from the norm at some point, though not necessarily at the time of diagnosis.

- **Immunologic disruption,** suggested by any of these three findings in blood tests:

  (1) Evidence of the *antiphospholipid antibody syndrome* (APS; in Great Britain, also known as Hughes syndrome), signaled by the presence of antibodies to a particular group of substances found in cell membranes, based on one of the following:

  (a) A false-positive reaction to the standard test for syphilis, persisting for at least six months and confirmed as false by the use of alternative testing methods.[1] This occurs in about 20 percent of those with lupus.

  (b) A positive test for lupus anticoagulant; this occurs in about 10 percent of those with lupus. A test for this antiphospholipid antibody is called the PTT, for partial thromboplastin time. Despite the word "anticoagulant," which seems to suggest that it prevents blood clotting, it's actually associated with an increased risk of the formation of dangerously obstructive blood clots.

  (c) An abnormal level of anticardiolipin antibodies (ACL); this is found, at one time or another, in perhaps one-third to one-half of lupus patients. Cardiolipin is a substance found in cells lining blood vessels.

  The antiphospholipid antibody syndrome affects perhaps 1–2 percent of the general population but a far higher percentage of lupus patients—so, while it is not by itself diagnostic of lupus, its presence is suggestive of *something* amiss immunologically. APS is a special concern in relation to pregnancy and is discussed in detail in Chapter 6.

  (2) An abnormally heightened level of anti-DNA, an antibody to DNA (deoxyribonucleic acid), particularly double-stranded DNA (dsDNA) or "native" DNA, the kind found within the nucleus of all human cells; this antibody is often called "anti-dsDNA." Anti-dsDNA is found in at least 50 percent of lupus patients at some time. Some researchers believe that the antibody to native DNA may be unique to lupus, making this assay a highly specific one, though not

particularly sensitive. (See the earlier explanation of sensitivity and specificity.)

DNA with another molecular structure, known as single-
stranded DNA (ssDNA), is also found in the bloodstream as
a result of the breakdown of old or damaged cells. Most lupus patients also have anti-ssDNA, but so do those with
rheumatoid arthritis and other connective-tissue disorders;
anti-ssDNA may be found, as well, in perfectly healthy
people.

(3) The presence of anti-Sm, another antibody. "Sm" is not a
medical abbreviation but stands for the name of the patient
in whom it was first identified; it is a nuclear protein. Anti-
Sm has been found in fewer than half of lupus patients (the
reported range is 30 to 40 percent), but, like anti-dsDNA, it
may be unique to lupus—a finding with low sensitivity but
high specificity.

- **High levels of antinuclear antibodies (ANA),** antibodies that
act indiscriminately against material from cell nuclei. They don't
actually invade cells but, rather, apparently react to a variety of
proteins that may be released when cells have been destroyed.

High ANA levels are suggestive of lupus, though not exclusive to lupus; they're also found in a number of other conditions,
including rheumatoid arthritis, liver disease, and some infections, as well as in those taking certain medications. The proportions of positive results vary, however—from at least 90 percent
(and perhaps very close to 100 percent) of lupus patients to
about 30 percent of people with rheumatoid arthritis and varying proportions of those with other connective-tissue disorders
and other diseases. They are also found in a small percentage of
healthy elderly people. ANA testing is thus highly sensitive, but
not specific.

The last two ACR criteria involve *antibodies*. You may be more familiar with the word in connection with infectious diseases, where
antibodies are viewed as highly desirable. They are developed by the

body in response to infection or to a vaccination in which infectious agents are deliberately introduced to evoke the manufacture of antibodies. Thereafter, those antibodies stand guard, ready to defend the body against that particular disease-causing agent. A substance that provokes the body's immune system to produce antibodies is called an *antigen*, since it stimulates production of an "anti" substance; antigens are usually composed of protein.

But in lupus, and in the other connective-tissue disorders, tissues of the patient's own body are somehow perceived as foreign invaders, like bacteria or viruses, and *they* act as antigens. ANA and the other antibodies mentioned in the diagnostic criteria, unlike our antibodies against polio, measles, or the flu, have been produced to do battle with the stuff of the body's own cells. They are *autoantibodies*, hence the characterization of lupus and the others as autoimmune disorders—conditions in which the body is primed to protect itself against itself.

Why should these substances from the patient's own body act as antigens? No one knows. But the antibody-provoking substances are not intact tissues and organs. Rather, they consist of cellular fragments that have somehow been released and have set off this autoreactive frenzy.

All cells die eventually; the body is constantly renewing and replacing itself, efficiently disposing of old, worn-out cellular material, with no disruption in the smooth running of the body as a whole. This normal process of preprogrammed cell death is called *apoptosis* (the name of this routine process is from two Greek roots meaning roughly "falling away"). Scientists exploring the origins of autoimmune disease now suspect that something may go awry during this normal ongoing process, something that triggers the abnormal autoreactive activity.

OTHER SIGNS, SYMPTOMS, AND TESTS

Although they are not currently on the list of official criteria, there are a number of other signs, symptoms, and test results that, if present with others, will lead an experienced specialist to consider the possibility that a patient may have lupus. Some are considered more significant than others. Among them are the following (the first three were formerly included in the official ACR diagnostic criteria but were later dropped):

- **Hair loss.** Rapidly occurring, unexplained loss of hair from the scalp. There are many possible causes of hair loss, ranging from mechanical stress to allergies and infections, and the physician will look for such alternative explanations. About a quarter of all lupus patients experience some degree of hair loss.
- **Raynaud's phenomenon.** Pain and color changes affecting the fingers—occasionally, the toes, nose, or ears—sometimes known as Raynaud's *syndrome* or *disease*. It can also occur alone, not in association with any other disorder.

  This condition is caused by vasospasm, spasm of small blood vessels that cuts off circulation. The cause is unknown. It is essentially identical to frostbite, although extreme cold isn't needed for it to occur; attacks, lasting minutes or hours, may also be triggered by other stimuli, including emotional stress. Raynaud's is sometimes referred to as the "red, white, and blue" phenomenon: The fingers or toes turn very pale, then blue, and these two stages are either preceded or, more often, followed by painful redness. Estimates of the proportion of those with lupus who suffer from Raynaud's have varied from fewer than 20 percent to 40 percent. See Chapter 5 for more about this condition.
- **A positive LE-cell test.** Sometimes referred to as "LE prep," the LE-cell test is a test for a unique sort of white blood cell that shows evidence of a phenomenon called aberrant phagocytosis. Certain white cells normally engage in phagocytosis, roughly translatable as "cell-eating," in which bacteria, body discards, and other cellular debris are disposed of; the LE cell is such a cell interrupted in the process of devouring nuclear core material from another white cell, after the latter has been attacked by a destructive agent called antideoxyribonucleoprotein antibody.

LE cells are found in an estimated 40 to 50 percent of lupus patients at one time or another, especially when the disease is active (lupus has a flare-and-subside pattern). Despite their name, however, LE cells aren't unique to lupus; the test is also positive in 5 to 10 percent of those with rheumatoid arthritis, and some common medications can also cause a positive LE-cell test in some people. The LE-cell test was dropped from the ACR criteria in 1997, and few rheumatologists now use it as a diagnostic tool.

- **Free DNA.** As noted, the antibodies in lupus are produced in response to encounters with the nuclear material of cells or specific components of that material. Unusually high levels of freely circulating DNA, which suggest high levels of cell destruction, while not specifically pointing to lupus, are highly suggestive of lupus.

- **High sedimentation rate.** The erythrocyte (red blood cell) sedimentation rate (ESR; often called the "sed rate") describes the sinking velocity of red cells within a quantity of drawn blood. The ESR tends to be elevated in most lupus patients with active disease—as well as in most rheumatoid arthritis patients and during the course of many infections, as well. A higher-than-normal ESR doesn't necessarily signify lupus—its specificity is *very* low—but it does indicate something amiss.

- **Other antibodies.** One of the possibilities mentioned in the ACR diagnostic criteria is an antibody against a substance called Sm. Sm is one of several substances collectively called extractable nuclear antigens, or ENAs; others include Ro, La (like Sm, named for the patients in whom they were first discovered; anti-Ro and anti-La are, for unknown reasons, often seen together), and RNP (ribonucleoprotein; anti-RNP is often seen with anti-Sm).[2] The specialist who suspects that a patient may have lupus will probably test for antibodies to all known ENAs.

About 15 percent of lupus patients have anti-La, while 30 to 40 percent have anti-Ro, and these antibodies are often accompanied by anti-Sm. Both anti-La and anti-Ro are even more highly associated with Sjögren's syndrome, another autoimmune condition that may "overlap" with lupus and is discussed in detail in a later chapter. Anti-Ro is often associated with marked photosensitivity. An estimated 40 to 45 percent of lupus patients have anti-RNP antibodies, which seem to be associated particularly with such symptoms as arthritis and Raynaud's phenomenon and with a low incidence of kidney involvement.

Most recently, rheumatologists have begun testing for anti-chromatin antibodies, antibodies specifically against the genetic material of the cell nucleus; it is believed that these antibodies may precede the appearance of anti-dsDNA and thus provide an early clue. Anti-chromatin antibodies have been found in about 70 percent of lupus patients and have relatively high specificity for lupus, although they have occasionally been found in rheumatoid arthritis and scleroderma.

By and large, the presence of one or more ENAs, especially anti-RNP, is often suggestive either of lupus or of *mixed connective tissue disease* (MCTD), a situation in which a patient appears to the rheumatologist to have lupus, *as well as* manifesting symptoms of at least one other of the autoimmune disorders. Often, though not invariably, the MCTD patient is less severely ill with either of the "overlapping" disorders than many patients with only one of them.

• **Serum complement.** The complement system, which is part of the body's overall defense operation, is a series of proteins that perform in conjunction with antigen-antibody activities.

When antibodies attack antigens, they lock in combat (imagine two tenacious wrestlers), forming entities called immune complexes, which cause local inflammation and a certain amount of injury. Immune complexes attract the complement-system components, which move in to destroy the membranes of the "enemy" cells by a number of techniques, including summoning phagocytes to the area, coating cell membranes with a substance phagocytes can "recognize," and producing solvents to destroy the membranes. It is this battling, with its frenetic activity, that causes the severe tissue damage, particularly in the kidneys, that can occur in lupus.

The total amount of complement in the body at any given moment is finite. Thus, if complement has been drawn to sites of immune complex activity, there will be lower-than-normal levels in the general circulation. In lupus, at least in active disease, serum complement levels are low. (This pattern is also helpful in monitoring treatment.)

- **Rheumatoid factor.** A procedure called a latex fixation test may reveal a particular antibody, called rheumatoid factor, found in 75 to 80 percent of rheumatoid arthritis patients. The test is also positive in about 15 percent of lupus patients, as well as in 25 to 40 percent of those with scleroderma or polymyositis; that is, the antibody is not highly specific, but it may signal connective-tissue disease of some sort.

- **False-positive AIDS test.** In a few instances, false-positive tests for infection with the human immunodeficiency virus (HIV), the cause of acquired immunodeficiency syndrome (AIDS), have occurred in individuals who later turned out to have not AIDS but lupus.

The most commonly used HIV screening test is the enzyme-linked immunosorbent assay, or ELISA, widely employed because it is inexpensive and easy to perform. Although the test is quite sensitive, it is not very specific, and false-positive results with ELISA are not uncommon. Other, more specific tests are available, notably the Western blot test, which is more costly and requires more expertise but which is used to confirm positive results on the ELISA test. In rare cases, even the Western blot test has been known to give a weak false-positive result in a lupus patient.

SORTING IT OUT

In medicine's past, syphilis was known as "the great imitator," because in its various stages, it can affect many parts of the body and can appear in many different and seemingly unrelated guises. Now, syphilis can be promptly treated in its earliest stage with antibiotics, and lupus has assumed the "great imitator" title.

Arriving at a definite diagnosis isn't easy, even with the use of laboratory tests, since there is significant overlap—either of symptoms or of actual illness—with other chronic disorders, especially those in the autoimmune family. We've mentioned rheumatoid arthritis, Sjögren's syndrome, and Raynaud's phenomenon. Another is Behçet's syndrome (named for the Turkish dermatologist Hulusi Behçet, who first described it in the 1930s), an autoimmune vasculitis that often involves mouth sores and skin lesions much like those seen in lupus. Others that frequently overlap are myositis, which features muscle inflammation, and fibromyalgia syndrome, evidenced chiefly by pain in muscles and connective tissues.

Lupus may even be confused with infectious ills. A number of them—including rubella, Lyme disease, and some strep infections— may be accompanied by arthritis-like symptoms.

Aside from the previously mentioned mixed connective tissue disease, there is another situation called—for want of a better term— *undifferentiated connective tissue disease* (UCTD). Here, the patient is clearly suffering from a disorder in the connective-tissue disease family, yet the combination of symptoms, signs, and laboratory test results are not fully consistent with the diagnostic criteria for lupus—*or* for any other related condition. Although a variety of results and observations may point strongly to lupus, or rheumatoid arthritis, or some other member of the group, no combination of them meets the criteria. Not *yet*, anyway.

If a definitive diagnosis cannot immediately be established—leaving the patient in the limbo of a UCTD "diagnosis"—the physician will usually want to follow the patient's course carefully, repeating certain tests or other diagnostic procedures at intervals, with both patient and physician on the alert for changes and new developments. Meanwhile, aches, pains, and other symptoms will be treated as they arise.

NOTES

1. "False-positive" suggests falsely that the patient has the disease being tested for. The false-positive suggestion of syphilis (which can also occur in other conditions, including acute hepatitis) is associated with a widely used screening test called the RPR (for rapid plasma reagin). Two other tests— the FTA-ABS (for fluorescent treponemal antibody absorption) or the TPI (for *Treponema pallidum* immobilization)—can be used to rule out syphilis.

2. Ro is also sometimes known as SS-A and La as SS-B, the designations they were given when first found, in patients with the condition called Sjögren's syndrome, which may exist alone and also affects some lupus patients. A person may have antibodies to Ro or La without having Sjögren's, however, so the Ro and La appellations are preferable.

CHAPTER

3

What Causes Lupus—Maybe

There is a kind of "lupus"—not *really* lupus, but a condition very much resembling lupus—for which a cause can often be singled out. That lupus-like syndrome, discussed in Chapter 12, is set off by a specific substance, usually a drug, and it departs when the culprit is withdrawn. But the cause of lupus itself is unknown—although there have been hints, suspicions, and many theories.

This much *is* known:

- Lupus is not transmissible—by sneeze, by cough, by touch, by sexual intercourse, by living or working with a lupus patient, or by any other known means. There is not the remotest suspicion that anyone has ever "caught" lupus from someone else. Although there may be an infectious agent or agents involved in lupus, it is not an agent that can carry the condition from one person to another, like the measles or flu virus or the bacteria that cause tuberculosis or syphilis.
- Lupus is not inherited, passed on from parent to child like the color of one's eyes or the shape of one's nose or a tendency to tallness. Although there may be a genetic factor involved in lupus, it does not act in a predictable manner, like a gene for

hemophilia or dwarfism. Nor is it related to some congenital anomaly, like the abnormal chromosome configuration in Down syndrome.

- Lupus is not induced by any identified environmental toxin. Although there may be an environmental substance involved in lupus, there is not a one-to-one correspondence as can be drawn, say, between asbestos and mesothelioma, or lead and brain damage.

- Nor, to round up other possibilities, has lupus been traced to the absence or presence of any specific vitamin, mineral, or other nutrient; to an overabundance or undersupply of any specific hormone, enzyme, or other substance produced by the body; or to allergy or other form of sensitivity—although it's possible that one or more of these phenomena may play a part.

Is this simply a matter of scientific curiosity? Does it matter, as long as therapies to cope with lupus and control its symptoms are available and improving? Yes, it does matter, because no ill has yet been *cured* without understanding the *cause*—whether that has turned out to be the presence of a bacterium, the absence of a crucial enzyme, or an assault by an environmental toxin. More important, once a cause is clearly established, the matter of *prevention* can be addressed.

Increasingly sophisticated technology is now enabling medical researchers to examine and understand the disease process, at the cellular level, in lupus and in the other autoimmune disorders. But understanding *what* is happening is not necessarily knowing *why*—or how the process might be halted, reversed, or prevented. We simply don't yet know what causes some people to become ill with lupus. There are only intriguing associations that seem to suggest, if not a provable cause, at least some sort of influence. Much current thinking holds that these factors likely interact to cause lupus, that two or even more must occur simultaneously. There are a number of interesting areas of study.

THE GENETIC CONNECTION

I have lupus, and so does my sister, although hers is very mild. We think our mother may have had it, too. We remember that when she was in her forties, she had a real bad time; she'd be exhausted, she'd have aches and pains and headaches. Nothing was ever diagnosed. I gather that years ago, lupus often wasn't even considered unless there was a butterfly rash and kidney disease.

Lupus doesn't run in families in the way that certain heritable diseases do. If someone in a family has Huntington's disease or cystic fibrosis, for example, the odds of it being passed along to the next generation can be mathematically calculated, because inheritance of these diseases follows a predictable pattern. Depending on whether each parent has the disease or carries a gene for it, the probabilities may range from 25 to 100 percent. There is no such specific gene, or formula, for lupus. Aside from the special, usually temporary condition called *neonatal lupus* (discussed in Chapter 6), there is only about a 5 percent chance of a person with lupus having a child who will eventually develop lupus.

Yet, there have been suggestions of more subtle genetic factors. Overall, about 20 percent of lupus patients have a first-degree relative (parent, child, or sibling) with *some* autoimmune disorder, which might be lupus but might be thyroid disease, insulin-dependent diabetes, rheumatoid arthritis, multiple sclerosis, or any of a number of other, less well-known conditions.

An additional 15 to 20 percent of lupus patients' close relatives, if their blood were thoroughly tested, would be found to have signs of immunologic aberration, such as antinuclear antibodies (ANA), although they have no autoimmune disease.

Another intriguing research area is that of twin concordance. Twins who share a characteristic are said to be concordant for that trait; if one has it and the other does not, they are discordant for it. In fraternal twins, who are dizygotic (originating from two separate fertilized egg cells) and are no more closely related than any two siblings of different ages, the likelihood that they will be concordant for lupus is a mere 2 to 5 percent.

But in identical (monozygotic) twins, who originated from a single fertilized egg cell and are genetically identical, much higher concordance has been reported, ranging in various studies from 24 to 57 percent. That certainly suggests that some hereditary factor is at work.

Still, the figure is not 100 percent—indeed, not even close. Clearly, having an identical twin with lupus doesn't mean that you will have lupus; clearly, there is not a single "lupus gene." Rather, the high degree of identical twin concordance suggests an inherited susceptibility; some additional factor(s) must be present, as well, for lupus to occur. Some researchers call this the "fertile soil" concept: The direct cause that triggers the development of lupus might be thought of as "seeds"; unless they're sprinkled on ground that offers the right growing conditions, the "fertile soil" of susceptibility, nothing will happen.

To further explore such factors, the National Institute of Environmental Health Sciences launched a search in the spring of 2003 for same-sex sibling pairs—both twins and close-in-age brother pairs and sister pairs—in which one sibling has a particular autoimmune/rheumatic disease and the other does not (that is, in considering causes, both sex and marked age differences are being eliminated from consideration). The institute hopes to enroll 400 families in the study, which will include patients with lupus in addition to those with rheumatoid arthritis, systemic sclerosis, and idiopathic inflammatory myopathy (an autoimmune muscle disease).

Another aspect of genetic study is what has come to be known as the HLA system. The letters stand for "human leukocyte antigen," so named because it was first found in leukocytes (white blood cells); later, it was found that a region on the sixth chromosome of every human cell contains genetic coding that controls a number of immunological responses, including the acceptance or rejection of transplanted tissue and organs. The name was nevertheless retained. (It is also known as the major histocompatibility complex or MHC; *histos* is Greek for "tissue.")

As scientists have studied this tiny but influential territory, they have pinpointed a variety of subregions—designated A, B, C, and so on—and, within those subregions, certain proteins that have been identified as genetic "markers"; like blood types, they are determined by heredity. HLA "typing" is now standard procedure in transplant surgery.

But these HLA markers indicate more than whether a person is likely to be compatible with another individual's kidney. The HLA region can apparently also reveal something about susceptibility to certain disorders.

The first such connection surfaced in the early 1970s, when researchers found that the HLA marker designated B27 turned up in 80 percent of those with ankylosing spondylitis, a disabling form of spinal arthritis which strikes mostly men and had been observed to recur in families; the marker was found in fewer than 10 percent of persons without the disease.

Since then, other HLA factors, especially those in the "D" subregion, have been associated with a variety of chronic problems. DR4, for example, has been linked with both rheumatoid arthritis and diabetes. And two closely associated DR markers have been found in lupus patients in statistically significant numbers.

Although results of various studies have not been completely consistent, DR3 has been found in 44 to 54 percent of those who have lupus, versus only 20 to 36 percent of those who do not; DR2 has been found in more than half of lupus patients, but in only about a quarter, or even fewer, of other individuals (DR2 has also been linked to multiple sclerosis). Overall, 75 to 85 percent of lupus patients have either DR2 or DR3 or both; that's true for fewer than half of those without the disease.

More recently, the "next-door" DQ subregion has been found to be even more closely associated with a number of the specific antibodies characteristic of lupus (see Chapter 2 for more about those). Those associations include DQ2, DQ6, or DQ8 with anti-DNA; DQ5 or DQ8 with anti-RNP; and a DQ6 subtype with anti-Sm (there's also an association of this antibody with DR4 and DR7). Lupus patients who have both DQ2 and DQ6 almost always have both anti-La and anti-Ro antibodies (and those with these two antibodies, interestingly, nearly always have DR4, as well). And DQ7 is linked with the antiphospholipid antibody syndrome (see Chapter 6).

Still another suggestion of a genetic component in lupus lies in its racial distribution. While lupus is doubtless underreported and firm figures are hard to come by, it's been estimated that in the United States, lupus strikes at least 1 in 700 women between the ages of 20 and 64. But among African American women in the same age group, the incidence is estimated to be about 1 in 245, nearly three times as high. Lupus is also more prevalent among both Asians and Native Americans than among whites, and some observers have noted higher prevalence among Hispanics. The changing demographics of the US population may mean changes in the prevalence of lupus as well.

There also appear to be slight differences in patterns of disease among ethnic groups. While patients in every group can and do experience all manifestations of lupus, African Americans and Asian Americans seem somewhat more likely to have more active disease; Hispanics are more likely to have heart or kidney involvement; and Caucasians are more likely to experience skin lesions and thrombocytopenia. There also seem to be some divergent disease patterns among groups of different Asian descent. (These are general population observations, not necessarily true of any individual.)

Another curious matter is the case of the anti-Ku antibody. The various antibodies mentioned in the discussion of diagnosis in Chapter 2 are found in lupus patients of all races, although anti-Sm and anti-RNP seem a bit more frequent among African Americans. One specific antibody (not noted in Chapter 2), designated anti-Ku, is found in a significant minority of African American patients with lupus but is quite rare in Americans of European descent. In one multicenter study reported in the ACR journal *Arthritis & Rheumatism* in 2001, anti-Ku was found in 12 percent of African American lupus patients but in none of the white patients in the study. The same antibody, interestingly, is strongly associated in the Japanese not with lupus but with a mixed syndrome combining facets of scleroderma and polymyositis.

A research project—ongoing at this writing—was launched in the late 1990s by the National Institute of Arthritis and Musculoskeletal and Skin Diseases (NIAMS), the agency within the National Institutes of Health that deals with the rheumatic disorders, to investigate the influence of ethnicity, including genetic factors, on the expression and impact of lupus in the various ethnic groups. The study, called LUpus in MInorities: NAture versus Nurture (LUMINA), includes several hundred lupus patients, aged 20 to 50, from the various groups and is a cooperative venture being conducted by researchers at the University of Alabama in Birmingham and University of Texas medical centers in Houston and Galveston. All aspects of the disease, from clinical attributes and psychosocial factors to genetics and antibodies, are being explored, including the apparent differences noted above.

SEX DISCRIMINATION

The fact that lupus strikes at least eight or nine times as many women as men might seem to suggest another heredity-related question. Could there be something about femaleness that predisposes one to lupus? Women have two X chromosomes, men one X and one Y. Might some genetic information on the X chromosome encourage lupus—something that's countered in most but not all cases by genetic information on the Y chromosome? Of course, that just raises more questions, including, what sort of message would be found on some Y chromosomes but not on others? And, of course, no "lupus gene" has ever been found, despite long and diligent searching, on an X chromosome or anywhere else.

How about hormones, then? The population of those with lupus is skewed not only by sex but by age as well. Lupus has been diagnosed in infants and nonagenarians, but the concentration of cases at onset is from the teens through the forties—that is, the reproductive years. During these years, the ratio of females to males among lupus patients is at least nine to one; some estimates have even run as high as fifteen to one. After age fifty, women patients still predominate, but the ratio drops to approximately two to one—and that's when the childbearing years are over, menopause occurs, and the general activity of the female hormones diminishes. Furthermore, a study of all the children and teenagers diagnosed with lupus over more than a decade at a major metropolitan children's hospital showed a dramatic spurt in new cases at ages eleven and twelve, the onset of puberty.

Might sex hormones play a role in lupus? If so, might one expect to find marked departures from normal hormone profiles in people with lupus? These questions have been studied, but the number of research subjects has been small and the findings inconclusive. More often than not, serum levels of the female hormone estradiol have been somewhat elevated, and those of the male hormone testosterone somewhat below average, in both male and female lupus patients. Still, the findings have not been fully consistent, and both higher- and lower-than-average levels of androgens (male hormones) and estrogens (female hormones) have been observed in both men and women (both sexes produce both; it's the proportion that counts).

There may be somewhat more significance in levels of another hormone, an adrenal androgen called dehydroepiandrosterone (DHEA), which appears to be notably lower in lupus patients of both sexes. DHEA is basically a precursor of *both* testosterone and estradiol, as well as a third hormone, the pregnancy-related hormone called progesterone. The significance of this observation is being further explored, and some feel that DHEA may have therapeutic potential (see Chapter 13).

The relationship of observed patterns of these sex hormones to levels of still other hormones—those produced by the pituitary, for example—is complex, but may offer answers to these puzzles, and is being further investigated. Preliminary reports attribute particular significance to abnormal levels of such hormones, especially that of prolactin (which plays a major role in enabling breast-feeding) in both male and female lupus patients; that phenomenon, too, is being explored.

There is a race of hybrid mice, known as NZB/NZW (they're native to New Zealand, and the line was developed by breeding black mice with white ones), that spontaneously develop an ailment striking in its resemblance to lupus in humans. They have been under study for more than four decades. In these mice, administration of estrogens has been found to accelerate the illness, and androgens have proved protective. Despite this correlation, exacerbation of an already existing illness doesn't mean that the same factor can also be cited as a cause. Nor does successful therapy in mice necessarily mean that similar therapy would be suitable for humans.

Some have suggested that the apparent significance of sex hormones in humans might be explained not by undersupply or oversupply but by how they're handled by the body. Parallels can be drawn with other conditions. Disease due to lack of a vitamin isn't always due to dietary deficiency, for example; sometimes, it's caused by inability to absorb or metabolize foods containing the nutrient. Many cases of diabetes are not caused by underproduction of insulin but by failure of the body to utilize it properly.

Indeed, one small study did find that lupus patients of both sexes metabolized (chemically broke down) estradiol, an estrogen, differently from a group of healthy volunteers. And another small study reported by rheumatologists in Russia and in France found increased activity in lupus patients (both male and female), compared to control subjects (healthy people used for comparison), of aromatase, an enzyme that converts circulating androgens to estrogens. Aromatase activity was especially elevated in patients with minimal disease activity; in those who were severely ill, aromatase levels decreased and were even lower than those in the healthy controls. The researchers weren't sure of the meaning of these findings, but it would appear to be a potentially fruitful path for future exploration.

How about the pattern of disease? Is lupus manifested differently in men and women? Not markedly, but one study reported in the early 1990s did turn up some minor variations. Among 64 percent of the women, almost two-thirds, arthritis was an early symptom; that was true for only 40 percent of the men. The men, on the other hand, were more likely than the women to have discoid lesions at the onset of the disease (17 percent versus only 1 percent).

Later on (the patients were followed up for an average of four and a half years), the men continued to be more likely than the women to have discoid lesions (20 percent versus 3 percent), while the women were more likely than the men to have arthritis (81 percent versus 60 percent) as well as the classic butterfly rash (52 percent versus 23 percent).

On the other hand, it must be noted that a second study, reported at about the same time, came up with no significant differences in symptoms between male and female patients. (The first study took place in Barcelona, the second in London. The numbers of patients were similar.)

Remember the question of identical twins, though. In such twins, with identical genetic patterns, there is higher concordance of lupus—but it's not 100 percent. So it is with the sexes: Far more women than men develop lupus, but the difference isn't 100 percent; some men *do* develop lupus. If hormones play a part, it's likely that there is some interplay, some mutual impact, involving an additional factor.

A QUESTION OF INFECTION?

The lack of total concordance among identical twins implies that there must be some other factor or factors. If one thirty-five-year-old woman has lupus, and her identical twin—with exactly the same genetic risk factors—does not, we have to conclude that the lupus patient has yet another risk factor, one that her twin does not. Logically, that must be something in her environment, something she has encountered that her sister has not. What might that be? Increasingly, the environmental factors that have come under suspicion have been viruses in general, and certain categories of viruses in particular.

Viruses are organisms consisting of a core of genetic material surrounded by a protein coat or shell. All viruses are classed generally as either riboviruses or deoxyviruses, depending on whether their cores consist of ribonucleic acid (RNA) or deoxyribonucleic acid (DNA). Each class includes a number of subgroups.

Among the RNA viruses are the myxoviruses, which have a special affinity for mucous membrane (*myxa* is Greek for "mucus") and include the influenza viruses; the related paramyxoviruses, which include the measles, mumps, and rubella viruses; the parainfluenza viruses, which typically cause colds in adults but more serious respiratory ills in infants; the reoviruses, which are not known—yet—to cause any specific diseases (they've been associated with minor ills such as mild gastrointestinal upsets, but no cause-and-effect relationship has been proved); and the retroviruses, of which more in a moment.

Over the years, a number of RNA viruses have come under suspicion as possible culprits, or at least aiders and abetters, in lupus. Quite a few researchers have reported significant proportions of lupus patients with antibodies to reoviruses; in one study, the figure was 55 percent, versus only 3 percent of controls. Some have found comparatively high levels of antibodies to various parainfluenza viruses (there are four known strains) among those with lupus. Many have linked lupus to high levels of antibodies to the paramyxoviruses, especially the measles virus. Still, these links have not proved completely consistent. Most recently, there has been growing attention paid to the subclass of RNA viruses known as retroviruses.

All viruses are essentially parasites, invading living tissue in order to thrive and multiply; they lurk, and reproduce, within the cells of their host. This mode of reproduction is one of the means by which viruses elude the usual antibiotics, which can easily seek out and destroy bacteria wandering the bloodstream. Antiviral drugs, thus far few in number, must rely on more sophisticated strategies that will vanquish infectious agents while sparing the host itself, typically by interfering in some way with the virus's reproductive process. Retroviruses are unique in employing an effective counterweapon, an enzyme called reverse transcriptase, which enables them to convert RNA to DNA and then slip into target cells virtually undetected. There, they may remain for a long period of time, even years, until some unknown signal activates them.

It has been known for quite some time that retroviruses are responsible for a number of malignancies in animals. It was not until 1981, however, that a retrovirus was found to cause a human illness, a rare form of leukemia; it was dubbed human T-cell lymphotropic virus, or HTLV, for its attraction to a class of white blood cells called lymphocytes, and particularly to a subclass of those called T cells. A second, similar virus, dubbed HTLV-2, was later identified and, still later, a third, labeled HTLV-3. The last proved *not* to be the cause of any sort of cancer. Rather, it has proved to be one of the most devastating agents of human disease ever discovered; it is now better known as HIV, human immunodeficiency virus, and it is the cause of the acquired immune deficiency syndrome—AIDS.

There have been a few hints that a retrovirus may be involved in lupus, and in a related disorder as well. Several years ago, two groups of researchers—at the University of Texas in San Antonio, and at the Pasteur Institute in Paris—announced that they had found antibodies to retroviral proteins in small groups of lupus patients, as well as in approximately 30 percent of a group of Sjögren's syndrome patients. HIV and other known human retroviruses were *not* present (the antibodies were not to those viruses, only to certain proteins). Could an unidentified retrovirus be associated with lupus? No one yet knows.

This intriguing discovery presents a particular puzzlement: If a retrovirus is involved in lupus, it is one that behaves very differently from the AIDS virus—in a contrary manner, in fact.

There are two main types of lymphocytes. One group, called B cells, produces immunoglobulins containing antigen-specific antibodies targeting specific foreign invaders. The second group is made up of the T cells. They comprise "helpers," which produce a variety of substances, collectively known as lymphokines (interferon is one), that actively repel infectious agents, and also function as "aides" to the B cells—marshaling phagocytes, for example, to clean up cellular debris; and "suppressors," which restrain inappropriate B-cell activity.

In AIDS, the immune system apparently falters because the primary cells depleted by HIV are the "helper" T cells. The result is that people with AIDS succumb to infections and other conditions normally fended off successfully (more than two-thirds of the deaths in AIDS are caused by lung infections).

In lupus, quite the opposite is true. There is a marked deficiency of "suppressor" T-cells, with an eight- to tenfold increase in the proliferation of antibody-producing B-cells—in lupus, referred to as *autoreactive* B cells. It appears that among those antibodies are some directed specifically against "young" T-cells that are in the process of developing into suppressors. Thus, these two retroviruses—assuming that there *is* a retrovirus involved in lupus—must behave very differently, with one killing off "helper" cells and the other depleting the population of "suppressor" cells.

Among the DNA viruses are, notably, the large family of adenoviruses, which are responsible for many childhood nose, throat, and eye infections (with age, we build some immunities); the poxviruses (smallpox and others); and the notorious herpesviruses. The adenoviruses and the poxviruses aren't suspected of any lupus connection. Interest has focused on the herpesviruses, in part because of their notoriety.

Once the herpesviruses move into the body, they take up permanent residence. They may emerge again and again to cause recurrent episodes of the same condition—like the herpes simplex viruses, which linger in skin and mucous membrane and cause cold sores, among other annoyances. Or they may trigger a completely different problem on subsequent appearances; the varicella-zoster virus—which causes chickenpox, retreats to nerve tissue, and causes shingles on reemergence—is the prime example. As the years go by, more and more of this nasty tribe (the family name comes from the Latin *herpes*, in turn from the Greek *herpeton*, "reptile," from *herpein*, "to creep") have been identified and numbered:

- HHV (for human herpesvirus) 1 and 2 are the two herpes simplex (HSV) types, which trigger cold sores, canker sores, and genital sores.
- HHV 3, the varicella-zoster virus or VZV, causes chickenpox (varicella) and, on reemergence, shingles (herpes zoster).
- HHV 4, lymphocryptovirus, also known as Epstein-Barr virus, is behind a number of ills varying geographically, including infectious mononucleosis in the United States and at least two types of cancer (chiefly in Africa and the Far East). It especially targets B lymphocytes.
- HHV 5, cytomegalovirus (CMV), can cause pneumonia and other infections, chiefly in those with impaired immune systems.
- HHV 6, roseola virus, was isolated only in the 1980s. Nine out of ten of us have encountered it at some time and will test positive for it. It causes the typically mild infection called roseola infantum—or sometimes exanthem subitum—in small children and, possibly, mild illness in adults; it has also been associated with more serious problems, including lung inflammations following bone marrow transplants.
- HHV 7 has no name of its own and is similar to, but distinct from, HHV 6; it may be a "co-factor" in roseola and may also be associated with an acute, not uncommon skin inflammation called pityriasis.
- HHV 8, rhadinovirus or Kaposi's sarcoma herpesvirus (KSHV), is believed responsible for a particular cancer seen in AIDS and has also been linked to a number of other conditions, including pulmonary hypertension and multiple myeloma (a kind of blood-cell cancer). It seems to strike only when immune defenses are down and, like HHV 4, singles out B lymphocytes.

Most of these have either been cleared, or have not been suspected, of a lupus connection. The exceptions are HHV 6 and, most recently, HHV 4.

Researchers reported in the 1990s on a study in which a group of lupus patients, a second group with rheumatoid arthritis, and a third group without autoimmune disease were tested for HHV 6 (roseola virus) infection. Remember that almost everyone has had this virus at some time and so would have antibodies to it. But *active infection* was found in 44 percent of the lupus patients, and in only 2.3 percent and 6 percent, respectively, of the other two groups. Interestingly, HHV 6 is also under suspicion in another autoimmune disorder, multiple sclerosis.

Several investigations have directed suspicions toward HHV 4, the Epstein-Barr virus (which has long been a suspect in fibromyalgia, as well, and has recently come under suspicion in childhood-onset multiple sclerosis). Two teams of investigators reported at a 2003 meeting of the American College of Rheumatology that they had found in groups of lupus patients, as compared with healthy subjects, elevated levels of Epstein-Barr virus (EBV) in one study and, in both, what the researchers called "altered" or "dysfunctional" T cells primed specifically to respond to that virus—that is, lymphocytes that had apparently been transformed by contact with the virus so as to behave abnormally.

It is likely that when the primary cause of lupus is found—and it *will* be found eventually—it will turn out to be a virus, whether a retrovirus, a herpesvirus, or some other type, that behaves in an unusual manner (or is *permitted* to behave in an unusual manner in some individuals, perhaps those with particular genetic characteristics).

There is, of course, the possibility that the development of lupus—as well as other autoimmune disorders—requires a combination of two or more infectious agents simultaneously attacking a genetically susceptible individual and setting off an unstoppable immune-system reaction. Perhaps the massive autoreactive activity in these conditions stems from a frenzied immune-system effort to stave off simultaneous acute infection by, say, a retrovirus and a herpesvirus. Such avenues remain to be explored.

OTHER ENVIRONMENTAL AGENTS?

One phenomenon suggesting some role for environmental factors is the coincidental occurrence of autoimmune disorders in pet owners and their pets. Although most diseases affect either animals or humans but not both, there are exceptions, including such viral infections as the infamous swine flu and equine encephalitis, and fungal infections like ringworm (the latter is easily caught by children from puppies and kittens).

> *I've had my symptoms for about five or six years, I guess, but I just got my lupus diagnosis a year and a half ago. And there's this weird coincidence. My cat, Teeny—she's now five years old—got sick when she was around six months old. The vet's diagnosis was autoimmune hemolytic anemia. She said, "This is very rare in cats, and it never comes back." She seemed to get better—and it came back a year later. It keeps coming back, like—well, like lupus flares. I can tell when they're coming on: She gets tired easily. She plays less. I'm sure she has joint pain; she gets mad when her hips are touched, and she won't let me hold her paws to trim her claws. The only thing that helps are corticosteroids. Now does that sound like lupus, or what? And is this just a coincidence? Or did we both catch something?*

Dogs, as the nation discovered in mid-1991, can have lupus, too. In May of that year, President George H. W. Bush received a diagnosis of Graves' disease, an autoimmune disorder of the thyroid gland. His wife, Barbara, has the same condition, diagnosed at the beginning of 1990. And in the summer of that year, the Bushes' springer spaniel, Millie, was found to have lupus.

This situation is, to put it mildly, extremely unusual. According to newspaper reports, the Bushes' physicians called the coincidence "bizarre," and a variety of experts were said to estimate the odds of a husband and wife both developing Graves' disease as ranging from 1 in 100,000 to 1 in 3 million—not to mention the odds of such a couple also having a dog afflicted with an autoimmune disease.

A common cause, perhaps? A virus? Some other infectious organism? Table scraps shared with Millie? Furniture, fixtures, or some other factor in the family wing of the White House?

There is some disagreement about whether autoimmune disease in cats can properly be termed lupus, although the signs and symptoms—anemia, fatigue, apparent joint and muscle discomfort—may mirror those in human (and canine) lupus.

There is no question about the existence of lupus in dogs, which was first described in 1965 and is now identified on the basis of the same diagnostic criteria as human lupus (and the diagnosis is just as difficult). The most prominent symptom is polyarthritis—involving many joints—which afflicts nine of ten animals with the disease. About 60 percent have skin or mucous membrane lesions, and almost two-thirds have kidney involvement. Treatment is very similar to that of human lupus, using many of the same drugs. As in humans, there is a flare-and-remission pattern. And in another parallel with the human disease, the typical skin lesions of canine lupus—which generally occur around the nose—are worsened by exposure to ultraviolet light.

But what of both people and their pets having autoimmune diseases? Has anyone undertaken a scientific study of this sort of phenomenon? Yes, on a small scale. A group of immunologists in England did so and reported the outcome in 1992 in the British medical journal *The Lancet*. Fifty lupus patients were randomly selected from the researchers' hospital register and asked about dog ownership; only pets that lived in the house with their owners were included in the study. All the dogs were apparently well. Blood tests were performed, and the results were compared with test results from a group of certified healthy animals that served as controls, as well as with test results from a group of dogs with a definite diagnosis, or at least marked evidence, of autoimmune disease.

As expected, significantly more anti-DNA antibodies were found in the dogs known to be ill than in the control animals—but the average for the lupus patients' dogs was even higher. Additionally, all the blood samples were subjected to serum protein electrophoresis testing, which reveals unusual levels of antibody-containing immunoglobulins; abnormal patterns were found in 33 percent of the patients' dogs and in 44 percent of the autoimmune-disease group but in none of the controls.

The study was a small one, and the results do not prove anything about the cause(s) of autoimmune disease in people, the cause(s) of autoimmune disease in dogs, or what they may have in common. The researchers cautiously concluded, however, that the findings "lend support" to the idea that "common environmental factors or transmissible agents" may play a role—and that further research along these lines would be worthwhile.

Whether or not lupus in people and lupus in pets may be triggered by shared environmental factors, aside from infectious agents, what might those factors be? Connections have been noted only in humans, and thus far, they are only tenuous statistical correlations. Investigators who make it their business to follow up such threads also warn of jumping to conclusions. Coincidence does happen, and researchers seeking causes and effects must ever beware of falling into the trap of *post hoc, ergo propter hoc*—literally, "after that, thus because of it," the assumption that, just because B happens to follow A, A is the cause of B. As the old song says, it ain't necessarily so.

Among the connections, possibly merely coincidental, that have been noted are the following:

- **Tobacco smoke.** It has been demonstrated that smoking can trigger flares in lupus and generally make the disease worse. Might it actually play a *causative* role? A Norwegian-American team reported in late 2003, after completing a study of more than 20,000 people, that smokers appeared to be 1.8 times (approaching twice) as likely to develop another autoimmune disease, multiple sclerosis, as nonsmokers. An apparent smoking connection has also been observed in autoimmune thyroiditis and possibly in Graves' disease. And most recently, an analysis of nine small lupus studies by rheumatologists at Harvard Medical School suggested that cigarette smoking may raise the risk of developing lupus by 50 percent; the investigators emphasized that only *current* smokers, not those who had quit, appeared affected, and they added that genetic factors, as well as other environmental exposures, could also play a part.

- **Local pollutants.** Higher-than-usual rates of particular diseases in certain geographical areas, generally termed "clusters," often give rise to speculation on the role of local phenomena—industrial or agricultural pollutants, for instance. A somewhat elevated occurrence of lupus in the vicinity of Nogales, Arizona, is one prominent example, reported in the mid-1990s. There were suggestions that exposure to pesticides and other industrial contaminants might be responsible. Investigations by the federal government (at the state's request), however, while confirming the higher local prevalence of lupus, could verify no connection with pollutants; evidence of exposure to certain chemical components of locally employed pesticides was found to be higher than the national average—but no higher in lupus patients than in anyone else. The reports didn't comment on the possibility that the toxins might have combined with some other (genetic?) factor to trigger autoimmune disease.

- **Drugs.** Many medications and other substances with which we may come into contact can trigger a temporary lupus-like syndrome—not really lupus, but a condition that exhibits many of the same characteristics as long as the substance is present (see Chapter 12). Indeed, according to the Lupus Foundation of America, more than seventy different drugs have been associated with such syndromes. None, however, has been proved to cause lupus itself.

4

The Main Lupus Meds

Lupus is a complex illness, more like a spectrum of diseases than a single one. It's multifaceted to start with and may be further complicated both by coexisting autoimmune diseases and, alas, by a constellation of other conditions that commonly attack lupus patients. While piling on pills never makes medical sense—and it's especially unwise in lupus—medications nevertheless are usually needed.

Drug treatment of lupus has progressed through three general stages over the past few decades. Roughly until the post–World War II period, around the midpoint of the twentieth century, the approach was what might kindly be called trial and error—or more bluntly, hit or miss. Little had been established as to potential risks or potential benefits. Among the many let's-try-it-and-see-if-it-works substances employed were gold (some forms of which *are* effective in rheumatoid arthritis), bismuth, liver extracts, and an array of vitamins.

Subsequently, a number of specific drugs were found to be truly helpful in various manifestations of lupus. Because their benefits were recognized before their range of hazards were fully realized, they came to be overused, in both dosage and duration of treatment, with the result that patients were sometimes made sicker by their medicine than by the malady the medicine was meant to allay. And since some medications may give rise to symptoms not unlike those of lupus itself, the temptation to heap drug upon drug was probably understandable in some cases.

Happily, there has been a reversal. The trend is now toward conservative treatment—meaning a stance in favor of administering or prescribing medications only when they are clearly needed and then only in the quantities necessary. Unfortunately, not all lupus patients, in all circumstances, are always so treated. It can't be observed too often that laboratory tests don't necessarily reflect a patient's actual state of health. Nevertheless, some of those who treat lupus seem to focus on the lab tests, "treating" the tests rather than treating the patient.

In fact, other-than-normal values on blood tests may even turn up in people who don't have lupus at all. When such test results occur in relatives of patients, they may suggest interesting possibilities regarding familial factors in the genesis of autoimmune diseases in general and lupus in particular. When they occur in persons who share a patient's home or workplace, they may set off intriguing speculation about environmental influences. But no one has ever suggested that those people should receive any treatment.

Patients themselves *may*, however, need drug therapy. And there are a number of medications that, when used appropriately, have proved consistently valuable in the treatment of lupus. But first, some basic cautions about medications generally.

Lupus patients may often be on a relatively complex medication regimen, including therapies for acute or chronic conditions *other* than lupus. Lupus itself, as well as some of the drug regimens needed to treat it, may predispose one to still other conditions needing treatment—and of course lupus patients are subject to all of the same illnesses, both acute and chronic, as the rest of the population. Moreover, the fatigue and emotional ups and downs that often accompany lupus can sometimes play havoc with memory and attention. For all these reasons, it's a very good idea to write down all medication dosages, schedules, and other particulars—including the name and phone number of the prescribing physician—so that no mistakes are made.

Be sure to establish and record *exactly* when and how medications should be taken—that is, time of day and relation to meals. Some medications should be taken with food, or a certain amount of time before or after eating, or on an empty stomach; some should not be taken with certain types of foods; some pills should not be taken with certain liquids. (And *none* should be taken with, or within two hours before or after, grapefruit juice, which can interfere with the breakdown of a broad assortment of drugs.) This kind of information does not necessarily appear on your medication's label, or even in the accompanying literature.

If you know you're among those lupus patients who are photosensitive, which means that sunlight can trigger rashes or other symptoms, let any physician or dentist prescribing for you know about that right away. Some drugs can intensify photosensitivity, and the doctor who is forewarned will select an alternative medication.

Similarly, let doctors know ahead of time about allergic or other reactions you've had in the past to any medications—rashes, stomach upsets, whatever. *Most* medications produce side effects, which may be physical, mental, or both and may be major or minor. Some of these effects are common, others uncommon or even rare—but these terms reflect only statistics, not predictions for any individual. Depending on the seriousness of the reaction, this may mean that you should not take a particular drug, that a class of drugs should be avoided, or simply that certain protective measures (against stomach irritation, for example) need to be taken.

Remember to keep your physician completely informed—about any unexpected symptoms (which may mean side effects, lupus activity, or something else entirely), about whether a new medication plan is working or not, about drugs prescribed by any other doctor. And let other doctors you may consult know exactly what drugs you're taking for lupus.

Always remember that all of the medications employed in the treatment of lupus—in fact, most medications that may be taken for most ills, whether prescription or nonprescription—can be extremely hazardous, and even fatal, to infants or toddlers who may ingest them accidentally. Small children have peculiar senses of taste and smell, are not particularly discriminating, and may gobble down lethal doses of even foul-tasting substances.

"Childproof" containers (which sometimes aren't, for a child with better-than-average dexterity) may not make sense for a patient with hand and finger joint involvement. If there are small children in your home, or if small children might visit your home, keep your medications completely out of possible reach, preferably under lock and key.

Therapies for the major related ills that may beset lupus patients, as well as some of the unwelcome complications, are discussed in the subsequent chapters. Here, we examine the four main families of medications currently used to treat lupus itself.

THE CORTICOSTEROIDS

Most prominent among current lupus medications are those known as *corticosteroids*. They will be prescribed for almost every lupus patient at some time, whether on a short- or long-term basis, and both their benefits and risks are many and complex. Like most medications, they have advantages and disadvantages—but with these drugs, the "ups" and the "downs" are perhaps more extreme. They have more than once been termed "double-edged swords."

Don't confuse this group of drugs—often referred to simply as "steroids" by physicians and patients alike—with another, widely publicized group of substances called by the same familiar name.

The term *steroid* is actually a catchall designation for an array of organic compounds; the name is based upon details of their chemical structure at the molecular level. Substances classed as steroids include, among others, cholesterol, bile acids, some vitamins, and many hormones; among the latter are testosterone and other androgens, as well as estrogens and some of the hormones produced by the adrenal glands.

You may have read or heard about the "steroids" used illicitly by (predominantly male) athletes and some teen-aged boys. The full name of those hormones is *anabolic-androgenic steroids.* They are synthetic testosterone derivatives, and they are taken for their skeletal-muscle-building (anabolic) effects; they are also masculinizing (androgenic), and as used by those young men (and even a few young women), they are extremely hazardous to health.

The drugs discussed here, the corticosteroids, while extremely potent, are *not* the same as the anabolic steroids and do not pose the perils of those testosterone derivatives. This family of agents are synthetic hormones resembling cortisol, a hormone produced by the cortex (outer layer) of the adrenal glands. They are not boosters of muscle or machismo. They do, however, have their own benefits and risks.

I had lupus but, in a way, I hadn't really "had" it. I'd had an episode of horrible joint pain for about 24 hours in my midtwenties. They couldn't figure it out, so they gave me all kinds of tests. I had the false-positive test for syphilis and "passed" enough other tests so the conclusion was that I definitely had lupus. But the symptoms went away as quickly as they'd arrived, and the specialist said, no matter what the blood tests said, as long as I wasn't sick, he wasn't going to load me up with any powerful drugs.

But six years later, that suddenly changed. By now, I was in my early thirties. I was managing an antiques shop, I was working 80-hour weeks, I was under a lot of stress in my personal life too, and then my mother, who had been living by herself since my father died, fell very seriously ill. Suddenly, I was really sick. My symptoms were mainly fatigue, low-grade fever, and painful joints, with swelling in my hands and feet. But I was so busy that it was three months before I saw my doctor—who of course sent me to a rheumatologist as soon as I mentioned that I'd been diagnosed with lupus. The rheumatologist confirmed that after the lovely remission, now, I really had it!

For the next year and a half, I took a bunch of different antiinflammatory pills, but they controlled my symptoms only slightly. I still had a lot of pain and terrible fatigue. My rheumatologist kept saying, "You should go on prednisone." But I didn't want to, because I'd heard about the side effects, mainly weight gain. And then a really weird thing happened to change my mind.

It was August, I was due for a two-week vacation, and I was planning a bike trip in France with a friend in early September. One day, I was sitting outside, and a caterpillar fell onto my leg. That night, I woke up with flaming welts. I called my dermatologist, who prescribed prednisone. The welts cleared up in one day; I don't think I was aware of it at the time—I was focusing on what was obviously an allergic reaction to the caterpillar sting—but I kind of felt better all over. I finished the prednisone prescription, and then I suddenly had excruciating joint pain! I was supposed to start packing for my trip that night.

I called my rheumatologist the next morning and said, "Okay, put me on prednisone. I'm not missing this trip." He started me on 10 milligrams. By that night, I could move. The next day, I was much better. I continued to improve, and I did go on the bike trip. When I got back, I went to see the rheumatologist. We gradually reduced my daily dose of the drug to 3 or 4 milligrams, with no problems.

Then, I got a case of stomach flu, and it kicked up everything all over again. My doctor had told me that infection, as well as stress, can kick off a flare-up of lupus. He was right. I was a basket case. We increased the dosage to 7 milligrams. It was a miracle. It was like a light went on. All of a sudden, I felt I was in control.

I've continued on prednisone—I haven't had any remission since then—generally on 5 milligrams; if I have bad symptoms, I go to 7 milligrams. If I take a trip, I take along both 5- and 1-milligram pills, so I'm prepared. I know every case of lupus is different, and I figured 7 was my magic number. But my doctor says it works for other patients, too, because that's the level the body manufactures normally. And I haven't had any of those bad side effects I was afraid of. Not only have I not gained weight, but I've managed to lose a few pounds through not being so stressed, eating right, and getting exercise.

Prednisone is one of the corticosteroids, also sometimes called glucocorticoids and often simply steroids for short. They are without doubt the drugs that have been found most useful in lupus. Prednisone is the most widely used, and there are a number of other versions, including prednisolone, methylprednisolone (Medrol), dexamethasone, triamcinolone, cortisone, hydrocortisone, and others. One may be more helpful than another for a particular patient.

These drugs play a part in therapy for a number of ills in addition to autoimmune disease, including, among others, respiratory distress in premature babies, certain cancers, asthma, migraine headaches, and severe allergic reactions. They are also used as replacement therapy in failure of the adrenals to produce the natural hormone, just as thyroid hormone or insulin is taken by patients who are not producing the needed levels of those substances.

In lupus and other autoimmune conditions, the corticosteroids have the effect of controlling symptoms, primarily by anti-inflammatory action and possibly by inhibiting the production of antibodies. They may be prescribed in low doses to be taken on a regular basis (maintenance dosage); taken in somewhat higher doses, for limited periods of time, to cope with flares of disease activity; or administered in huge amounts, often by injection, to deal with major crises such as deteriorating kidney function.

It's important to note that the chief action of steroids is to counter inflammation. Inflammation may also be a symptom of active bacterial or viral infection. Lupus patients are no less susceptible to infections than anyone else, of course, and while steroids suppress symptoms, they are not antibacterial or antiviral drugs and will do nothing to banish any infectious agents that may be present. Indeed, steroids can dangerously conceal such infections by doing what doctors call *masking* symptoms—and can, under some circumstances, actually reactivate or exacerbate certain *latent* infections, including tuberculosis and some fungal respiratory infections such as coccidioidomycosis ("valley fever"). Thus, before steroids are given, a physician will consider and rule out the possibility of an infection for which an antibiotic or other drug is needed.

A dose of 6 or 7 milligrams does approximate the body's usual secretion. But many patients require higher dosages to meet their needs. For some, a maintenance dosage may be 10 milligrams, 15 milligrams, or some other quantity.

> *A month or two after I started on prednisone, my periods started getting really weird. They're not exactly periods anymore. I get all the feelings like a period coming on, which with me is usually a little bit of bloating and maybe feeling kind of moody, but then no real period—just some light spotting for a couple of days, and that's it. It was a little scary. I called my doctor, and he explained it was just a side effect of the prednisone and said not to worry about it.*

Unfortunately, the corticosteroids can have a number of serious side effects, typically related to long-term administration and/or high dosages, so that under most circumstances, quantities will be kept as low as is feasible, and the drug will be gradually tapered off entirely if possible.

Among the possible adverse effects are weight gain; increased susceptibility to infection and/or masking of symptoms of infection (as noted above); slowed healing of injuries; easy bruising; unusual hair growth; cataracts; precipitation or worsening of diabetes mellitus, with elevated blood sugar levels; amenorrhea (absence of menstruation) or menstrual irregularity; coronary artery disease (possibly related to increased levels of lipids—cholesterol and related troublemakers); aggravation of peptic ulcer (generally considered a contraindication for these drugs); facial swelling ("moon face"); diminished bone mineral density, with development of osteoporosis; elevated blood pressure and lipid levels, raising the risk of heart and vascular disease; sleep problems; mood swings or mental disturbances[1]; reactivation of latent tuberculosis (persons with positive skin tests for TB should receive prophylactic anti-TB drugs if they must take corticosteroids); precipitation of glaucoma-like pressure buildup within the eyeball; and facial rashes that can be confused (but not by an experienced rheumatologist or dermatologist) with the rash of lupus itself.

Bear in mind that the foregoing is simply a list of well-known effects and that they're related, in general, to dosage and to duration of therapy. A particular individual may experience many, few, or even no side effects at all (though the last is rare). But there is one basic physiological impact that occurs consistently in everyone who takes these steroids.

That impact stems from the fact that the steroids suppress production by the pituitary gland of adrenocorticotrophic hormone (ACTH), the normal function of which is stimulation of cortisol production by the adrenal glands. This happens because the circulating hormone results in a "cortisol unneeded" message to the pituitary. Because ACTH production is highest between 4 A.M. and 8 A.M., corticosteroids taken in the evening can suppress it totally, while taking the drug in the morning, or dividing the daily dosage and taking portions at different times of day, can minimize the effect. If a steroid is prescribed for you, be sure to discuss the schedule with your physician.

> About a year and a half ago, I noticed that my urine was a funny color, like weak tea, and I called my rheumatologist in a panic. I was sent to a radiologist for a sonogram, and I also had a lot of blood tests and 24-hour urine tests. They apparently showed a lot of hematuria and proteinuria. They finally did a renal biopsy—that's where they actually take a sample of your kidney—and it confirmed that I had nephritis, which is kidney inflammation. I had prednisone pulse therapy, which is three days of 1000 milligrams per day, intravenously. I had it again a month later and again three months after that, and that seemed to resolve it. Now I go every three months for urine tests, and I take prednisone orally; I started with 20 milligrams on alternate days, and I now take 15 milligrams on alternate days.

With the shorter-acting steroids—prominently, prednisone and methylprednisolone—alternate-day therapy, taking the medication every other day rather than daily, is believed to be helpful in decreasing side effects that are due to suppression of normal hormone production. This is not true for some other drugs in the corticosteroid family, such as dexamethasone and triamcinolone, which persist in the body for several days.

After withdrawal of long-term corticosteroid therapy, meaning several weeks or more, there is an extended period of hormonal imbalance, with a deficiency of the natural adrenal hormone. (The condition in which adrenal failure to produce the hormone is the main problem is called *Addison's disease*. The temporary situation we're referring to here is sometimes known as "secondary Addison's disease.") Cortisol's normal function is helping the body withstand sudden, massive physical stress. During corticosteroid therapy and for at least a year thereafter, serious injury or surgery calls for prompt steroid supplementation, because a higher-than-normal level is needed under these circumstances, and the body will be unable to provide it.

Because of the increased susceptibility to infection, anyone taking steroids should be sure to have all appropriate immunizations. For adults, that means flu vaccine (plus pneumonia vaccine and any other precautions your physician advises). For children, that means the routine schedule of childhood immunizations, plus flu vaccine and possibly other special precautions; see Chapter 11 for further discussion.

A comment on the question of weight gain: Many patients find it to be a problem, while for others, it's a fear that doesn't materialize. Corticosteroids can cause some fluid retention, particularly if there is any effect on kidney function, but the resulting gain is very minimal. To a degree, the pattern of fat distribution on the body may also change. Significant weight gain, though, is mostly a matter of increased appetite. It's possible—though not necessarily easy—to overcome that with effort and determination.

The matter of steroids' promoting osteoporosis, with increased bone fragility, also deserves further comment. While the best-known consequences of persistent osteoporosis are wrist and hip fractures, the less dramatic fractures—compression fractures of the vertebrae, the bones in the spinal column—are actually a more critical threat to health. As the vertebral column is compressed, the lungs are compromised; for each collapse of a thoracic vertebra—one of those in the part of the column backing the rib cage, between the neck and the hipbones—there is a 9 percent diminution of lung capacity.

Thus, for the sake of both bones *and* breath, preventing osteoporosis *and* safeguarding lung function are vital. Take the advice in Chapter 7 to heart, with special attention to regular exercise, which will also help to counter the muscle weakness sometimes seen with long-term steroid therapy. And take steps to protect your lungs, as well: Avail yourself of flu vaccine, as well as pneumonia vaccine if your doctor so advises; stay out of polluted air and away from folks with respiratory infections; and don't even *think* about smoking.

Few of the systemic effects noted here apply in normal use of the corticosteroid creams and ointments—some can be purchased over the counter, without prescription—that are used to treat skin conditions. They are also less likely to occur with inhaled steroids, which are used to treat such conditions as asthma.

THE ANTIMALARIALS

Fatigue and general achiness have always been my main problems. Our vacation last summer was really awful. We went to a resort in New York State, and we'd planned to do all kinds of things, but we ended up just staying in the lodge the whole time. Then I went on Plaquenil. Since it kicked in, I've been doing much better.

Rashes used to drive me crazy—not just that famous butterfly rash but rashes all over. But Plaquenil really solved that problem. My rheumatologist told me it might take about six weeks to start working—and it did, almost to the day.

The antimalarials—drugs originally used in the treatment of malaria—were the first of the specific agents found helpful for lupus, and they are still employed; they've been in widespread use since the late 1940s. Quinine—the classic antimalarial—had been tried experimentally in lupus as early as the 1890s, and some related drugs enjoyed favorable reports a generation later, in the 1920s, when it was found that they seemed to be effective in clearing up cutaneous lesions associated with lupus.

Now, a number of quinine derivatives, known collectively as antimalarials, are used—notably, chloroquine (Aralen), hydroxychloroquine (Plaquenil), and quinacrine (Atabrine). They're helpful not only for the skin but for joint manifestations and fatigue as well. Some studies have also suggested that for some patients, continuing antimalarial therapy, particularly with hydroxychloroquine, may reduce the frequency and severity of disease flares. Patients should be aware that six to eight weeks or more—sometimes as long as ten or twelve weeks—may go by before the benefits of antimalarial drugs are evident.

> I was taking chloroquine until just recently. I went to the eye doctor, and he said he thought he saw changes. He sent me to a second eye specialist, and that doctor discovered that I had chloroquine retinopathy—even though I have 20/20 vision, and I'm not aware of any problems when I'm reading, or out walking, or driving. They find this through something called field of vision tests. The medication had to be stopped, before it got any worse. My doctor always kept telling me to go for checkups; I should have gone sooner.

Like all drugs, the antimalarials may have side effects, including scaly rashes and stomach upsets. These relatively common complaints affect only a minority of patients, perhaps one in five, at least with hydroxychloroquine, the most widely prescribed of the group—although lupus patients who tend to suffer from exposure to sunlight should be aware that these drugs may also lead to heightened photo-sensitivity. Physicians have generally been concerned about possible effects of the antimalarials on a developing fetus, and some feel that antimalarials are best discontinued well in advance of a contemplated pregnancy—although recent limited studies suggest that hydroxy-chloroquine may be safe. (For further discussion of drugs and preg-nancy, see Chapter 6.) With these drugs, though, the most worrisome impact is on the eyes.

A number of reversible effects involve the cornea, the transparent membrane covering the pupil at the front of the eyeball. Deposition of drug in this area may result in blurred vision when the medication is started and "halo" radiation around lights later on. This has not been seen with quinacrine—but with quinacrine, corneal edema (swelling) can occur, due to fluid accumulation. Slight yellowing may occur, so faint as not to be visible to the patient. Corneal anesthesia, in which the ability to feel pain is deadened, may occur with any of these drugs; that could prove dangerous in case of accidental injury or overexposure to sunlight. All of the foregoing effects disappear once the medication has been discontinued.

More serious is an irreversible condition involving the retina, the area at the back of the eyeball where images are focused and from which they are relayed to the brain by the optic nerve. It is called mac-ular retinopathy; it involves pigment deposits and is apparently related to both drug dosage and the degree of individual photosensitivity, which may, as noted, be increased by the drug itself. And the damage may progress for a time even after the drug is discontinued, so prompt discovery of any hint of trouble is crucial.

The risk of this toxic reaction seems to be higher with chloroquine than with the other members of the family, but patients taking *any* of these drugs should take four precautions:

1. Always wear sunglasses—preferably not only in bright sunlight but even when the sun is not shining and, if possible, indoors as well as out, especially if there may be exposure to fluorescent or

halogen lights. Be sure the glasses are of high quality and that they bar ultraviolet light.

2. Even when wearing sunglasses, avoid direct exposure to unshielded fluorescent or halogen lights, as well as to midday sunlight.

3. Have your eyes thoroughly examined by an ophthalmologist—a physician specializing in the eyes—before you start taking the drug (to establish a "baseline"). This examination should include visual field testing.

4. Have ophthalmologic examinations at regular intervals thereafter, so that the drug can be promptly stopped if there is any sign of retinal injury. This examination is vital, since the retinal deterioration is symptomless. Discuss the frequency of these checkups with your rheumatologist *and* your ophthalmologist; the question is related to several variables—including the specific drug and dosage, your size (dosage per pound of body weight is relevant), and duration of therapy—and intervals may range from several months to one year. These drugs have a long half-life (they remain in the body for some time), so continued eye exams may be advised for a number of months after cessation of the medication.

In addition to the corneal yellowing, be aware that quinacrine can also cause yellowing of the skin and a deep yellow tinge to the urine—sometimes causing undue alarm because of confusion with signs of hepatitis. Quinacrine can also cause an extremely unpleasant reaction in combination with alcohol, much like that of disulfiram (Antabuse), an agent used in the treatment of alcohol abuse.

And for the sake of completeness, we should add that, rarely, the use of antimalarials may lead to slight hearing loss. The effect occurs so seldom that hearing tests, unlike eye examinations, are not routinely advised.

By and large, most rheumatologists feel that the safest of the antimalarials, and the least likely to cause critical irreversible side effects, is probably hydroxychloroquine.

The antimalarials may have one incidental "side effect" that's highly beneficial: They may lower levels of the lipids (cholesterol and kin) that can clog arteries and promote coronary heart disease. Prednisone, a corticosteroid, can raise those levels, and adding an antimalarial may be protective.

THE NSAIDS

There is a large group of medications frequently used in rheumatoid arthritis and used by most of us at one time or another to relieve many types of discomfort. They are often used in lupus and other rheumatoid/arthritic diseases, as well. They are classed as nonsteroidal anti-inflammatory drugs—NSAIDs (pronounced "*en*-sades") for short—which simply means that they act against inflammation, as corticosteroids do, but are not steroids.

Some NSAIDs, such as aspirin and ibuprofen (Advil, Motrin, Nuprin), are available over the drugstore counter without a prescription; many others are not. (If you wonder why another major over-the-counter pain reliever, acetaminophen (paracetamol in the UK)—sold under such brand names as Datril, Liquiprin, Tempra, and Tylenol—isn't listed: Although it is at least as widely used as aspirin to relieve minor aches and pains and reduce fever, it does not have any significant anti-inflammatory action and hence is not useful in conditions where inflammation is the major problem.)

Aspirin and other drugs related to it are known as salicylates ("aspirin" was once a trade name for what is chemically acetylsalicylic acid), and they are sometimes helpful in lupus when the chief complaint is joint pain. The dosages, however, are higher than those the labels recommend for the usual purposes, and they are taken on a regular schedule rather than simply in response to discomfort.

Be warned that the salicylates, despite their widespread availability and use, are *not* innocuous drugs, especially in lupus. Take them only on your physician's advice, and follow your doctor's recommendations for quantities and timing. The salicylates may also sometimes be useful as preventive therapy in Raynaud's phenomenon (see Chapter 5) and in patients who are at high risk for developing blood clots.

A vast array of nonsalicylate NSAIDs are also available, chiefly by prescription but some in forms and dosages available over the counter. A partial list (in addition to ibuprofen) includes ibuprofen's cousins fenoprofen (Nalfon) and ketoprofen (Orudis); piroxicam (Feldene), meloxicam (Mobic), nabumetone (Relafen), tolmetin (Tolectin), naproxen (Naprosyn, Anaprox, Aleve), sulindac (Clinoril), etodolac (Lodine), diclofenac (Voltaren), and ketorolac (Toradol).

It sometimes seems, thumbing through the medical journals, that a new variation or formulation is introduced almost monthly. There is some validity to the seemingly infinite numbers, however, since some seem to work better than others for different people—so that if one doesn't seem to be effective, or ceases to be effective, the physician and patient have many others from which to choose.

Unacceptable side effects can also dictate discontinuing a particular drug. With the NSAIDs, a common problem, particularly with the salicylates, is gastrointestinal irritation; with long-term use of the drugs, ulcers may develop. Aspirin is available in buffered and other forms to diminish such reactions, and many of the prescription products introduced in recent years have been formulated specifically to avoid the possibility of such irritation. (Some NSAIDs have been combined with antacids under new brand names.) If you are taking an NSAID, your doctor may suggest antacids, or a protective anti-ulcer medication may be prescribed to prevent problems. And even if your doctor hasn't advised use of an antacid, *always* take NSAIDs with food or milk.

Another not-uncommon, dosage-related side effect, particularly with salicylates, may be ringing in the ears (medically called tinnitus), although those who experience it are in a distinct minority. Headache and fatigue are among other occasional reactions to NSAIDs, as are rashes, bronchial spasm, or other manifestations of allergy (persons allergic to aspirin may have similar reactions to some other NSAIDs). There are cross-allergies among the nonsalicylates, as well. Some of the prescription products may have even more serious adverse effects, among them impairment of kidney function, exacerbation of hypertension, anemia, liver disease, and blood-count abnormalities; not all are safe for use during pregnancy.

In the 1990s, a new category of prescription NSAID was introduced and extensively promoted within the medical community and to the public as an effective new kind of pain reliever—for arthritic pain, in particular—with the specific claim that it offered more protection against gastrointestinal irritation. These NSAIDs, like their predecessors, are useful additions to the list of analgesic/anti-inflammatory drugs. They are not, contrary to some gushing news reports at the time of their introduction, "superdrugs."

These newer NSAIDs act a little differently than their precedents, most of which perform by blocking an enzyme active in the inflammation process. The enzyme, cyclooxygenase, exists in two forms, and the earlier NSAIDs block them both to varying degrees. The new drugs selectively block only the second form of that substance and are categorized chemically as cyclooxygenase-2 ("cox-2") inhibitors, familiarly known as "coxibs." Thus far, three have been approved by the US Food and Drug Administration (FDA) for use in the United States: celecoxib (Celebrex), rofecoxib (Vioxx), and valdecoxib (Bextra); a fourth, etoricoxib (Arcoxia), is in trial use at this writing.

In long-term therapeutic trials performed with the coxibs, their ability to offer increased gastrointestinal protection has been confirmed. A significant number of people are allergic to them, however, and they have demonstrated cross-sensitivity with sulfa drugs (that is, someone allergic to one may be allergic to the other). In general, benefits and problems with the two groups of drugs are similar, except that the earlier NSAIDs unquestionably have greater potential to trigger more gastrointestinal irritation and bleeding (because cox-1, inhibited by those drugs, apparently exerts some protective effect), and the same anticoagulant effect also guards against clots, which the selective cox-2 inhibitors don't.

It must be reemphasized that despite their wide availability and genuine usefulness, the NSAIDs are not innocuous drugs. All NSAIDs, including the coxibs, may cause unwanted reactions, including gastrointestinal irritation. All NSAIDs can also adversely impact the nervous system, the liver, the skin, the kidneys, and (except for the coxibs) platelet function, in addition to triggering serious allergic reactions in susceptible persons. They may also interact in unpredictable ways with a vast number of other drugs, either increasing or decreasing the effects of those drugs.

Following a safety data review of both prescription and over-the-counter NSAIDs, the FDA issued a 2004 consumer risk-factors warning of circumstances that could set the scene for potential trouble. The list included the following factors: concomitant use of steroids, anticoagulants, alcohol, or other NSAIDs; advanced age; a history of gastrointestinal sensitivity or bleeding; underlying kidney disease; such chronic conditions as hypertension, diabetes, or congestive heart failure; and taking more of the drug than specified by the label (unless so instructed by a physician).

Be sure that your doctor knows *everything* you're taking. And any unexpected symptoms, however mild, or any worsening of prior symptoms that may occur while you are taking any drug should be reported to your physician without delay.

THE IMMUNOSUPPRESSANTS

The corticosteroids, discussed earlier, might be referred to as immunosuppressants, since they act in part by quelling immune-system activity. But the kinds of drugs generally meant by this term are the agents used to prevent the rejection phenomenon in organ transplants; that is, they suppress the immune system that normally—and desirably—acts to reject foreign agents invading the body. These drugs also interfere with the proliferation of quickly multiplying cells and so are used to treat some malignant growths. The rationale for their use in lupus is their ability to reduce the ranks of B cells that are producing antibodies.

Prominent among those that have been used to treat lupus are methotrexate (Folex, Mexate, Rheumatrex), azathioprine (Imuran), cyclophosphamide (Cytoxan), cyclosporine (Neoral, Sandimmune), and mycophenolate mofetil or MMF (CellCept).

Methotrexate, which is used fairly extensively in rheumatoid arthritis, has been found to be occasionally helpful in lupus. It has been associated with reemergence of the varicella-zoster virus (which causes shingles). It may harm a developing fetus and should not be taken by women who are, or may become, pregnant; after cessation of methotrexate therapy, it's best to wait at least three months before becoming pregnant.

Azathioprine and cyclophosphamide are the two immunosuppressants that have been used longest in the treatment of lupus, specifically in dealing with such major threats as critical kidney involvement. In many series of clinical trials throughout the past two decades, cyclophosphamide has been found to be by far the more effective—especially in rescuing threatened kidney function—and is the one of this class most likely to be called on when heavy-duty therapy is indicated.

Cyclophosphamide is sometimes used alone, sometimes in combination with prednisone or methylprednisolone, and it may be given either orally or intravenously. Often the latter involves *pulse therapy*, relatively high doses given by intravenous injection at specific intervals (of days, weeks, or months). In either case, some experimentation may be needed to establish the ideal form and frequency of therapy for the individual. The combination of cyclophosphamide and corticosteroid has been particularly successful in inducing lengthy lupus remissions.

Because these drugs are so powerful, they are administered—whether orally or intravenously—very, very cautiously and with constant monitoring. They are employed because they are destroyers. The destruction can, and indeed does, easily encompass more than the targeted cells—resulting in "side effects" that can range from slight to severe.

Since their prime action is suppression of the immune system, they lower resistance to infection. Serious effects of this nature are more likely with intravenous administration, but "minor" infections—including shingles and urinary-tract infections—have been known to occur even with oral cyclophosphamide. Among other documented consequences are nausea and vomiting, temporary hair loss, impaired liver function, anemia, a raised risk of osteoporosis, bone-marrow suppression with resultant anemia, oral candida infection ("thrush"), ovarian failure, hemorrhagic cystitis (bladder inflammation), sterility (which is dose-related and irreversible), and in rare cases, certain cancers.

The adverse effects don't necessarily mean that the therapy must cease. A change in the regimen, such as lowered dosage, can prevent or diminish the difficulties while maintaining benefits. Monitoring during therapy must include frequent blood counts, and of course, prompt reporting of adverse reactions is crucial.

One exception is a relatively uncommon condition—it affects 1 in about 300 people—in which, due to a genetic enzyme deficiency affecting metabolization of the drug, azathioprine is absolutely contraindicated due to potential bone-marrow toxicity. A test for the deficiency is available and should be performed prior to azathioprine therapy.

Mycophenolate mofetil (MMF) is the most recent addition to the immunosuppressants. This relatively new drug, which has a heartening track record in kidney transplants, has been undergoing extensive clinical trials in lupus patients for several years. It seems to offer significant advantages over earlier agents, apparently stemming from its ability to act a bit more selectively, targeting anti-dsDNA antibodies and hyperactive B cells in particular.

Thus far, researchers comparing MMF with cyclophosphamide report gratifying diminutions in devastating side effects while performing at least as effectively to keep lupus activity under control. Fewer adverse effects means not only fewer actual threats to the patient's well-being but diminished discomfort—discomfort that can sometimes be acute enough that the patient insists on stopping the therapy.

Several such promising trials were recounted at a 2003 scientific meeting of the American College of Rheumatology by researchers at medical centers in London and New York. The reported results were consistently favorable, with both a higher proportion of remissions and markedly lower incidence of serious adverse effects among the patients given MMF. At this writing, further long-term studies are being undertaken to determine the drug's usefulness over the long haul and to establish such key facts as optimal length of treatment and the drug's lasting ability to prevent relapse. Meanwhile, many rheumatologists have already turned to MMF in preference to the older immunosuppressants.

NOTES

1. If you have previously had psychiatric problems—or there is any family history of psychiatric problems—it is imperative that you mention this to your physician *before* you take one of these medications. The steroids that have been most often associated with adverse mental effects are hydrocortisone, dexamethasone, and prednisone, and the effects are often dosage-related.

CHAPTER

5

Nine Lupus-Connected Conditions

Lupus patients are, of course, prey to all the illnesses that beset people who don't have lupus, and it's outside the scope of this book to cover them all; a few have been touched on in other chapters. There are, however, several conditions that tend to strike those with lupus with unusual frequency. Some of these conditions "overlap" lupus in the autoimmune disorders spectrum; in other cases, lupus—or its treatment—renders patients particularly susceptible to certain conditions.

Two of those conditions, the antiphospholipid antibody syndrome and premature osteoporosis, are discussed separately; see Chapters 6 and 7. This chapter examines some significant others.

RAYNAUD'S PHENOMENON

In an earlier chapter, we mentioned some signs and symptoms that aren't—or aren't any longer—among the American College of Rheumatology's official lupus diagnostic criteria but are nevertheless "red flags" for experienced rheumatologists; among them is Raynaud's phenomenon (sometimes called Raynaud's syndrome or disease).

First described by the French physician Maurice Raynaud in the 1860s, this condition may affect from 5 to 10 percent of the general population, somewhat more women than men (for women, the figure may approach 20 percent). Among lupus patients, an estimated 20 to 40 percent suffer from Raynaud's. (It's even more common among people with scleroderma, another autoimmune disease, afflicting 85 to 95 percent; it appears to be one of the earliest symptoms.) It is also sometimes associated with a variety of other problems, including other connective-tissue disorders, carpal tunnel syndrome, and individual reactions to a variety of medications. Physicians may speak of Raynaud's as "primary" when it occurs by itself, "secondary" when it's associated with a connective-tissue disease or another condition.

Raynaud's affects circulation to the body's extremities—usually the fingers, less commonly the toes (rarely, the earlobes or tip of the nose), so that they become numb and discolored, as if frostbitten; sometimes the skin, as in actual frostbite, may even crack. An attack may last only a few minutes or may persist for several hours. It may come on not only in cold weather (although low temperatures exacerbate the problem) but under other stressful conditions as well, which may vary with the individual. Often, it's termed the "red, white, and blue" phenomenon, since there may be a sequence of extreme paleness followed by a bluish tone, and these may be preceded—or, more often, followed—by redness. The red stage is typically the most painful.

The cause of Raynaud's is sudden vasospasm, spasmodic constriction of arterioles (the smallest arteries), resulting in a cut-off of peripheral circulation. (The similarity of the mechanism to that causing chest pain when coronary arteries are blocked has earned Raynaud's the nickname "angina of the fingertips.") Raynaud's is actually an exaggerated version of a normal physiological response to extreme cold, in which the circulatory system curtails blood flow to the body's perimeter to conserve heat and assure maintenance of the body's core temperature. Some lupus patients who suffer from both migraine headaches and Raynaud's episodes have found a temporal correlation between the two.

In the past, not much could be done beyond quitting smoking (which exacerbates the condition) and taking sensible home measures—and in many cases, that's sufficient. Raynaud's patients often find that wearing two layers—wool gloves under heavy mittens—or battery-operated heated gloves in winter can be helpful, along with avoiding cold outdoor weather. People who have Raynaud's are advised to stay as warm as possible generally, with layered clothing preferred, and to always wear a hat in cold weather, since the scalp is a major route of heat loss. Even in summer, attacks can be triggered by handling cold drinks (and refrigerated or frozen foods any time of year), as well as by air conditioning. Avoiding emotionally stressful situations can also be helpful in preventing attacks.

In addition to these practical measures that can be taken by the patient, prescription medicines are now available. Several medications that act to relax and dilate blood vessels have proved helpful. A class of drugs called calcium channel blockers, originally introduced for the treatment of coronary heart disease, has been found particularly beneficial in Raynaud's, decreasing both the frequency and severity of attacks in about two-thirds of patients. These drugs may variously take oral (to be swallowed) and sublingual (under-the-tongue) forms. Patients who have found regular oral administration either ineffective or intolerable due to side effects often find that the sublingual form, used shortly before exposure to cold, can prevent an attack and is free of side effects. Many physicians suggest, too, that those subject to Raynaud's attacks take baby aspirin regularly as a prophylactic measure.

SJÖGREN'S SYNDROME

About 5 percent of those with lupus also suffer from Sjögren's syndrome, another autoimmune condition, involving extreme dryness in certain areas due to dysfunction of various moisture-producing glands, prominently the salivary and lacrimal (tear) glands; it's sometimes called sicca syndrome, from the Latin for "dry." It was first recognized as a distinct disorder in the 1930s by the Swedish ophthalmologist Henrik Sjögren (*Sjö-* is pronounced "show").

The syndrome also occurs in people who do not have lupus or any other associated disease—it's often then called "primary" Sjögren's—

and may be associated with dry skin generally, as well as with inflammation in various other parts of the body. About 90 percent of those who have primary Sjögren's are women; more than 60 percent have anti-La antibodies and over 90 percent have anti-Ro, but in lupus patients who also have Sjögren's, the proportions are somewhat lower. (These antibodies are further discussed in other chapters; see the index.)

Diagnosis of Sjögren's, differentiating the syndrome from other conditions that can cause many of the same symptoms, is established by specific procedures, focusing chiefly on the eyes and mouth. They may include, in addition to physical examination, Schirmer tests, which assess tear-gland function; slit-lamp examination, which detects eye dryness and inflammation; salivary gland biopsy (very small glands inside the lower lip are used); and a variety of blood tests, including analysis of antibody patterns. Diagnosis may still be elusive; according to the National Institute of Arthritis and Musculoskeletal and Skin Diseases—the branch of NIH that deals with the rheumatic/ autoimmune disorders—establishing a diagnosis has been known to take two years and occasionally as many as eight.

The chief ocular symptom is usually a sensation of "something in the eye"; some describe the sensation as "burning" or "gritty." There may also be redness and itching and other discomfort. A decrease in saliva leads to extreme dryness of the mouth, with difficulty in chewing and swallowing, constant thirst, and possibly soreness and cracking in and around the mouth and lips.

The medical label for the eye condition is *keratoconjunctivitis sicca*; *kerato-* refers to the cornea, *conjunctiva* is the medical term for the mucous membranes around the eye, and the *-itis* suffix indicates inflammation. There are a number of products available for relief, including "artificial tears." Most of the artificial-tears products—which must be used regularly, not just when there's marked discomfort—contain preservatives, to which some people are allergic, with the result that the condition is aggravated rather than relieved; a few products without preservatives are also available.

In 2003, the FDA approved cyclosporine in a special low-concentration ophthalmic emulsion (Restasis) for topical treatment of this problem. The drug, a powerful immunosuppressant, has been used systemically since 1980 to stave off rejection of major organ transplants. This dilute formulation, however, acts only locally and is reported to be helpful, safe, and without significant adverse effects (occasional transient "stinging" sensations on application have been reported by a small number of patients).

Many over-the-counter products are promoted for the relief of eye dryness and general irritation, promising above all to banish unsightly redness. Those drugs, called vasoconstrictors, are *not* intended for this condition; in Sjögren's, they will only create further dryness and discomfort.

Too-low humidity can further irritate dry eyes, so a humidifier may help. Avoid smoke and other airborne irritants, including strong winds. Use eye cosmetics sparingly (if at all), being careful to keep them away from sensitive mucous membranes, and use mascara only on the tips of lashes.

It is also possible for the tear ducts to be plugged so as to retain moisture, and many patients have found that this procedure has brought relief when no other measures have helped. It must be performed by a qualified ophthalmologist.

For mouth dryness, medically termed *xerostomia* (Greek for "dry mouth"), there are "artificial saliva" sprays; sugarless lozenges are often suggested, too. Two oral prescription drugs, pilocarpine (Salagen) and cevimeline (Evoxac), are also FDA-approved for treatment of xerostomia caused by Sjögren's.

Steps should be taken to prevent serious dental problems, since one function of saliva is to help wash away plaque, the invisible bacterial film that forms constantly on the teeth and precipitates cavities and periodontal disease. Regular dental visits are very important, as is scrupulous at-home tooth care, including plaque control (use a soft-bristled toothbrush and an anti-plaque fluoride toothpaste and rinse, and floss daily). Avoid candy and other sugar-heavy foods and soft drinks; stick to sugar-free chewing gum. You might also talk to your dentist about topical fluoride applications that will help provide further resistance to cavities.

Sometimes, mouth and/or eye dryness is accompanied by uncomfortable nasal dryness, as well. Try one of the several brands of saline nasal mists that come in spray bottles. Don't confuse these products—which are also effective for the nasal stuffiness accompanying a cold—with decongestant sprays; the salines are not medicated, can be used as often as desired, and will not cause the "rebound" stuffiness often seen with the decongestants.

In a few women, Sjögren's may affect the lubricating glands of the vagina, making sexual intercourse extremely painful. The solution is to use a lubricant—preferably a water-soluble type such as KY Jelly or Replens, since oil-based products such as petroleum jelly can be absorbed and are capable of causing circulatory complications. Avoid use of other, unneeded vaginal products that could add to irritation.

LIBMAN-SACKS ENDOCARDITIS

Another eponymic condition, affecting an estimated 10 to 20 percent of lupus patients, was named for Emanuel Libman and Benjamin Sacks, the two American physicians who published a description of it in 1923. In Libman-Sacks endocarditis ("inflammation inside the heart"), also known as verrucous endocarditis, tiny wart-like growths develop on the valves between chambers of the heart (*verruca* is Latin for "wart"). Most of those with this condition are positive for antiphospholipid antibodies (see Chapter 6).

Libman-Sacks endocarditis may be suspected if the physician detects a heart sound called an *organic murmur* (there are many, many kinds of heart murmurs), which signals some structural abnormality. The presence of the valve lesions can then be detected by echocardiography, a technique that employs sound waves to create a visual image of the interior of the heart. In most cases, the lesions cause no serious problems unless they become infected.

An infection of Libman-Sacks lesions, known as subacute bacterial endocarditis, can occur as a result of dental treatment, when bacteria—prominently, streptococci—may easily slip into the bloodstream and find their way to the heart. If you have Libman-Sacks lesions, it's wise to take prophylactic antibiotics before and after any dental procedure.

The antibiotic—usually amoxicillin, or another member of the penicillin family, or erythromycin in cases of penicillin allergy—is taken prophylactically before, and again a few hours after, the dental treatment, the exact times depending on the drug. Preferably, put your dentist and your rheumatologist in touch with each other, so they can discuss the best preventive strategy for you.

Dental procedures are of particular concern because the mouth happens to be a hotbed of bacteria, and most people visit their dentists fairly regularly. Other, less frequent procedures that could conceivably cause a break in mucous membrane and send bacteria into the bloodstream call for similar precautions; they include gynecological procedures such as Pap smears, as well as gastrointestinal probes such as sigmoidoscopy and colonoscopy.

Symptoms of infection of Libman-Sacks lesions consist mainly of initial fever followed by signs of heart failure, including irregular heartbeat and difficulty in breathing. It is a medical emergency and is life-threatening unless promptly treated with intravenous antibiotics.

AVASCULAR NECROSIS

In addition to the painful arthritis that afflicts so many people with lupus, another joint problem may arise in a significant minority of lupus patients; in various studies, the incidence has ranged from 5 percent to as high as 40 percent.

The condition is *avascular necrosis* (AVN)—also called *aseptic* or *atraumatic* or *ischemic* necrosis—of bone, or *osteonecrosis*. All of these terms describe facets of the condition. *Osteo* signifies bone, and *necrosis* denotes the death of tissue. *Aseptic* and *atraumatic* tell us that it's not due to either bacterial infection or injury; *avascular* that it's related to diminished blood supply; and *ischemia* is the medical term for anemia (a dearth of red blood cells, hence disrupted delivery of oxygen) due to obstruction of the blood supply to the affected area.

The cause is not well understood. Doctors long thought that AVN of bone in lupus patients was connected only with long-term corticosteroid treatment, but such treatment is actually associated with only about 35 percent of the cases. Some affected lupus patients have had extensive treatment with immunosuppressants; still others have had neither kind of therapy.

Statistically, other factors associated with high risk of AVN include a history of arthritis or other joint disease; conditions involving abnormal hemoglobin, such as sickle-cell disease; and an array of predispositions to circulatory problems, including smoking, high blood lipids, and diabetes. High lipid levels, in particular, appear to pose a major risk. Aggressive lowering of these risks may help to prevent the problem, and the prophylactic use of statins (cholesterol-lowering drugs) is becoming routine for patients who appear to be at high risk for AVN. Excessive use of alcohol is also believed to add to the risk.

Theoretically, any joint can be affected by osteonecrosis, but weight-bearing joints are most frequently involved. By far the most common is the hip, and the affected site is the head of the femur, the thighbone. The second most often affected joint is the knee, and the third is the shoulder. In most, but not all, cases, only one joint is affected.

Pain during use of the joint is the initial symptom; sometimes the pain may at first not be felt in the joint itself but is referred to a nearby area—in the case of a hip, the groin, the buttock, or even the knee. Later, there is pain while the joint is at rest, as well. Some time may go by, from months to as long as five years, before the damage is detectable on X ray, but other techniques, such as computerized tomography (CT) scans and magnetic resonance imaging (MRI), may confirm the condition earlier and should be used if there are symptoms but X rays show no departures from normal.

If AVN of bone is not treated, it will progress and will eventually cause serious dysfunction of the joint, with high risk of joint collapse and fracture. Conservative treatment—medications to lower lipids that create blood-vessel blockage, pain relievers, reduced weight bearing—has generally not worked well. The sole exception has been the shoulder joint, where a program of special physical therapy, focusing on muscle strengthening, has been successful in many cases.

With other joints, the first-choice treatment is a surgical procedure called core decompression. In this operation, a small core of tissue is extracted from within the ischemic (blood-deprived) area of the bone, serving two purposes. It relieves pressure on the microcirculation in the problem area, stimulating formation of new capillaries and healthy bone; and the extracted tissue is analyzed to confirm the diagnosis. The technique, which has been in use since the mid-1970s, is often successful in staving off progress of the necrosis and postponing the necessity for major surgery.

Once osteonecrosis has progressed far enough to be evident on X ray, core decompression is no longer a recourse. Total replacement of the affected joint may become necessary eventually, especially in the case of a constantly weight-bearing joint such as the hip or knee; it may be the only possibility if diagnosis has come too late for decompression, or even if decompression has been performed but failed to stay the progress of the condition. (Other surgical options, such as bone grafting, are actually more complex; they are not yet proven effective and are still the subject of clinical study.)

Great strides have been made in joint surgery, technically termed arthroplasty, in recent years. The first operations to replace the ball-and-socket joint of the hip were performed in the early 1960s, and this was the first joint-replacement surgery to be pronounced an unqualified success. The complicated hinge joint of the knee posed greater technical challenges, but those challenges have also now been met successfully. By 2003, approximately 170,000 hip replacements and more than 200,000 knee replacements were being performed in the United States each year.

I've had avascular necrosis of the hip, which was bad enough. I had a core decompression about five years ago, and so far, it's working, although the orthopedist warned me that I might still end up needing a joint replacement eventually.

After that, I developed another problem: I've severed tendons like they were spaghetti, including the tendons in both of my thumbs, one of them twice. The latest was a patellar tendon in my knee. It happens with very simple things; with one of the thumbs, I was just picking up a bag of oranges! I've had more surgeries than anybody I know.

Many lupus patients have suffered from what they often describe as "tearing" or "severing" of tendons connected with various joints; it's technically called *tendon rupture*. There are no published statistics on its incidence, but it's quite common. The culprit is a form of avascular necrosis—that is, deterioration of the tissue due to compromised blood supply. As with AVN of bone, it's not clear if it stems mainly from various therapies or from lupus-associated medical conditions; the cause is probably multifactorial. In some cases, there appears to be an association with ciprofloxacin (Cipro), an antibiotic often prescribed for urinary-tract and other infections, and it may be wise to desist from physical stresses (such as strenuous workouts) while on such therapy.

The tendon—which need not be associated with a weight-bearing joint—becomes frayed and can rupture easily, with little or no physical strain involved. Probably the most common site is a finger (or, depending on the tendon involved, two adjacent fingers). The tendon rupture causes an abrupt finger drop, and the victim may sometimes fear that a sort of minor stroke has occurred—but of course only that one tendon is affected, not an entire limb or side of the body, as in a stroke.

Repair of a ruptured tendon requires surgery.

TWO BLOOD DEFICITS

Major deficits in two crucial kinds of blood cells are often found in lupus patients.

Anemia is a broad term simply meaning a deficiency of red blood cells, not specifying the cause of that shortage. It can be caused by blood loss, for example, as a result of injury or surgery, or by internal bleeding resulting from a peptic ulcer (or stomach lining irritated by aspirin or other drugs). Prolonged, uncontrolled inflammation can also cause anemia, by disrupting the body's processing of iron, which is needed for the production of new red cells.

Another type of anemia is termed *hemolytic*, a word coined from two Greek ones that translate as "blood destruction." In the normal course of events, our bodies constantly produce new cells and discard old ones. An individual red blood cell lives for about four months and is ultimately sequestered and destroyed by the spleen; in hemolytic anemia, red cells are disposed of prematurely, after a time as short as two weeks. Many things can trigger hemolytic anemia, including toxins, bacteria, and drugs.

Anemia is not unusual in lupus and affects about 50 percent of patients to one degree or another. The most common kind is *autoimmune hemolytic anemia*, in which antibodies produced by the body attack its own red cells. Prednisone is usually effective, but not always. When it is not, splenectomy, surgical removal of the spleen, may be necessary. Blood transfusion may also be needed when anemia is severe.

Immune thrombocytopenia (ITP) may also arise in lupus (it can also occur independently); the causative mechanism is similar to that of autoimmune hemolytic anemia. Thrombocytopenia is a deficiency of thrombocytes, also called platelets, the blood cells that are necessary for normal clotting. Symptoms of a shortage may include nosebleeds, gums that bleed easily, or petechiae—small, spontaneous "bruises" that signal tiny hemorrhages in the skin. Sometimes a clue to physicians of the possible existence of ITP can be persistent postoperative or post-injury bleeding problems. Again, prednisone—sometimes combined with hydroxychloroquine (Plaquenil)—may remedy this condition, but in some cases, splenectomy is needed.

Removal of the spleen, which may be necessary in some other conditions as well, generally causes no ill effects, and its normal tasks are assumed by the liver and lymph nodes. The one adverse effect is that after splenectomy, an individual is more susceptible to pneumococcal infection (infection with *Streptococcus pneumoniae*, the most prominent bacterial cause of pneumonia), as well as salmonella infection; immunization is therefore urged for those who have had splenectomies. The levels of protective (antibacterial) antibody should be checked after vaccination and at intervals thereafter, since a decline over time has been reported in some lupus patients.

RECURRENT SHINGLES

> I thought it was hives. It's always on my rear end. You can feel it starting, tingling; within two hours, there are these eruptions the size of a dime or bigger. I never had a handle on what caused it. Then, I happened to be at my gynecologist's near the end of one episode, and I mentioned it. He took one look and said, "That's shingles." He prescribed acyclovir, which cleared it up within three days.

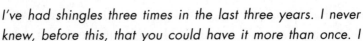

> I've had shingles three times in the last three years. I never knew, before this, that you could have it more than once. I guess it's because of the prednisone.

Steroids do disrupt the immune system, and recurrent shingles is not uncommon among lupus patients, assuming they have had chickenpox, which is caused by the same virus. That virus is one of the singularly unpleasant family of herpesviruses that have been proved or are suspected to be connected with illnesses ranging from cold sores to cancers (different conditions, different viruses) and share a particularly nasty characteristic: The herpesviruses trigger one kind of trouble when they first arrive; then they linger silently and ominously within the body, biding their time, until something—often a fall in the body's immune defenses triggered by illness or by therapy for an illness—offers an opportunity for them to reemerge, to cause the same condition, or one completely *different* from the original.

Chickenpox and shingles are the popular names for varicella and herpes zoster, and the virus responsible for both is known as the varicella-zoster virus, or VZV; it is also labeled HHV 3, ranked third in the list of eight human herpesviruses thus far clearly identified at this writing. (Numbers 1 and 2 are the familiar herpes simplex viruses that cause canker sores, cold sores, and genital herpes.)

An initial infection with VZV causes chickenpox. The virus, like other herpesviruses, then remains in the body—emerging, when circumstances are opportune, to trigger an episode of shingles, a usually painful (but sometimes, instead, intensely itchy) blistery skin eruption that typically occurs somewhere on the trunk (although it may appear anywhere, including the face), in a pattern following the nerves where the virus lurks between appearances. A person can have shingles *only* if he or she has previously had chickenpox; it occurs only as a reactivation, not as an initial infection. Most people will suffer shingles only once—although, theoretically, they *could* experience repeated episodes, as lupus patients often do. An episode may last for days, weeks, or even months.

A vaccine to prevent shingles has been under study since early 2000 in a nationwide clinical trial co-sponsored by the National Institute of Allergy and Infectious Diseases and the Department of Veterans Affairs. The double-blind trial (subjects were randomly assigned to receive either the real vaccine or an inert placebo, and the researchers didn't know who received which), enlisting nearly 40,000 subjects, ended in late 2003; the results were being analyzed as this book went to press.

The vaccine, a variant of the chickenpox vaccine (that vaccine has been routinely administered to children since the late 1990s), may or may not prove effective. Meanwhile, acyclovir and several other antiviral drugs can be used to treat shingles. Acyclovir is usually given orally for shingles (the drug is also available in intravenous and topical forms). At this writing, it has not been proved safe in pregnancy, although there have been no reports of adverse effects.

Anyone who has shingles should avoid close contact with pregnant women who have never had chickenpox, since chickenpox—that is, initial VZV infection—poses possible risks of complications to both mother and child.

Following an episode of shingles, some 10 percent of patients (the figure has been higher in some studies) may experience a lingering, acutely painful condition called *postherpetic neuralgia* (a medical term meaning "nerve pain"). The pain has been variously described as aching, burning, and/or exquisite sensitivity to the slightest touch. It appears to occur more often among those patients who are older (over the age of sixty) and/or have not received antiviral therapy for the shingles; those who have had the most widespread skin lesions and the most severe pain with shingles itself also seem to be more susceptible to this persistent aftereffect. Treatment is no different from that for any neuralgia or other intense pain; see Chapter 8.

FIBROMYALGIA

> I've been diagnosed with both lupus and fibromyalgia, and it's not only painful but confusing. At times, I don't know which one is acting up!

The rheumatic disease most recently recognized as a distinct disorder, with official descriptive/diagnostic guidelines, by the American College of Rheumatology is *fibromyalgia*, sometimes referred to as the fibromyalgia "syndrome," or FMS. The medical term is a combination of *fibro-*, referring to fiber or connective tissues; *my-*, a combining form from the Greek *mys*, "muscle"; and another combining form from the Greek *algos*, "pain". In short, the name means pain involving connective tissues and muscles—although there are typically other accompanying symptoms. It appears to be essentially the same condition generally labeled "chronic fatigue syndrome" a generation ago and various other names prior to that.

To say that this condition has been misunderstood is a gross understatement. The chief features are, indeed, pain and fatigue, which are of course subjective symptoms rather than objectively observable signs, and it often received (and sometimes still receives) curt dismissal by some physicians as being evidence of a vivid imagination, emotional disturbance, or deliberate malingering.

Uncanny consistency in particular symptoms, however, led to the acceptance of fibromyalgia as a distinct disorder by the late 1980s, and the ACR criteria were established in 1990; they include a history of widespread pain ("widespread" has a precise meaning in relation to areas of the body), as well as the presence of pain in at least eleven of eighteen specific "tender points." Rheumatologists also look for other key characteristics of the syndrome, apart from the official criteria, including disturbed sleep, whether in the form of insomnia or of "ineffective" sleep that, while of normal span, somehow fails to refresh and restore strength and energy; worsening of pain in the morning; and the aforementioned persistent fatigue.

Other signs and symptoms have also been reported in the years since FMS was officially recognized, although firm statistics reflecting their prevalence are few. Fibromyalgia patients may be aware of difficulty concentrating (it should be noted that studies have *not* demonstrated any intellectual deficits or abnormalities). There seems to be a higher-than-average incidence of certain other problems among FMS patients, including migraine headaches (and also ordinary tension headaches) and, according to some studies, depression, anxiety disorders, hearing and vision difficulties, and heart-valve abnormalities. A few small studies have suggested unusual variations in hormonal and other biochemical patterns. About one in six also suffers from Raynaud's phenomenon, discussed earlier in this chapter.

Perhaps most important, firm confirmation of experienced pain came in a 2002 report, in the ACR journal *Arthritis & Rheumatism*, of a brain-imaging study using a cutting-edge kind of visualization called functional MRI. The study compared a group of fibromyalgia patients and a similar group without the disease and found clear evidence of a distinct difference in sensory processing—what the researchers described as "a neurobiological amplification of their pain signals." In short, the patients aren't imagining things; they're *hurting*. The cause of this detectable functional difference is not yet known.

Although fibromyalgia, like the other conditions discussed in this chapter, may occur alone—and is estimated to afflict at least 3.5 million Americans—it's a frequent concomitant of several of the other connective-tissue diseases; probably at least one-third of those suffering from other connective-tissue disorders, including lupus, have overlapping fibromyalgia. The ratio of women to men is about seven or eight to one. And like lupus itself, fibromyalgia may mimic a number of other conditions, whether chronic or acute. Before confirming the FMS diagnosis, the physician must carefully test for, and exclude, problems sharing some of the same symptoms, including infections, malignancies, glandular dysfunctions, and other rheumatic diseases with similar symptoms.

The cause of fibromyalgia, as with the other disorders in the family of connective-tissue disorders, is not known. Some believe that it stems from some sort of alteration in muscle metabolism or a dysfunction in the nerves transmitting pain sensation. As with those other disorders, much speculation has focused on predisposition/susceptibility coupled with an environmental trigger, possibly an infectious agent. There is mounting evidence of familial, probably genetic, predisposition; at the 2003 scientific meeting of the ACR, several groups of investigators reported finding aggregates of FMS and/or FMS-related characteristics, such as aberrant pain thresholds and sensitivities and mood disorders, among family members.

As to precipitating agents: One suspect is the Epstein-Barr virus, one of the notorious human herpesvirus family (it's also known as HHV 4). Another is Lyme disease. Physicians at Tufts University reported in the early 1990s that they had seen fibromyalgia associated with Lyme disease in 8 percent of a series of patients with that tick-borne infection (the cause is a bacterium called a spirochete); although the Lyme disease itself was successfully treated in these patients, antibiotics had no effect on the fibromyalgia. Indeed, researchers at an ACR scientific meeting said that in one study of nearly one hundred patients thought to have Lyme disease, the vast majority were in fact suffering from FMS.

Treatment for fibromyalgia varies with, and is aimed at relieving, the individual patient's symptoms; no single drug or even class of drugs has been found to be consistently effective, and therapy may be a matter of trial and error until physician and patient see improvement. Unlike lupus, FMS does not respond to steroids, immunosuppressants, or antimalarials (and therefore it's important to distinguish this condition from a flare-up of lupus itself). NSAIDs (discussed in Chapter 4) may sometimes prove helpful, at least temporarily, as may muscle relaxants. More potent antipain medications, notably the synthetic narcotics called opioids, seem to be of some benefit in some patients but not in others (several researchers have raised the possibility that there are subcategories of fibromyalgia that differ in significant ways)—and, of course, raise concerns of dependency.

The most helpful drugs are often antidepressants, some of which appear to also possess important pain-relieving properties. They include, notably, the tricyclic amitriptyline (Elavil), as well as the newer types such as selective serotonin reuptake inhibitors (SSRIs). The doses used are generally markedly lower than those used to treat clinical depression. Again, there is marked variation in effectiveness among patients. At this writing, a multicenter study is in progress, under the auspices of the National Institute of Arthritis and Musculoskeletal and Skin Diseases (NIAMS), evaluating another agent, gabapentin (Neurontin), an antiseizure medication that has also been found valuable in treating the acute pain of various neuralgias.

Thus far, the firmest therapeutic conclusions physicians have reached about fibromyalgia are non-pharmacological—that is, not relating to medications. Likely to worsen FMS are very cold and/or very humid weather, undue physical or mental stress, and either too much or, conversely, too little physical activity. Likely to help in relieving pain and discomfort are warm, dry weather; hot baths and showers; and a program of regular, moderate exercise (such as cycling or swimming, especially in a warmed pool). If you suffer from stubborn FMS, you might also discuss with your doctor the possibility of physical therapy (a therapist can also prescribe helpful routines to be performed at home) or professional massage treatments; acupuncture has also been found to be sometimes helpful, and your physician may be able to refer you to a trained, licensed practitioner.

PULMONARY HYPERTENSION

Most of us have been taught the basic difference between the two main types of blood vessels: Those called *arteries* distribute freshly oxygenated blood from the heart to all of the body's tissues and organs; the *veins* make the return trip, carrying a stream of "used," oxygen-depleted blood, laden with discards and cellular debris. But there is also a second, smaller and separate, extremely crucial circulation; it consists of the pulmonary artery, which receives waste-laden blood from the heart and conveys it to the lungs, and the pulmonary vein, which returns oxygen-rich blood to the heart. A condition of elevated pressure confined to this small but crucial subsystem is called *pulmonary hypertension*.

Pulmonary hypertension is a major threat to well-being—indeed, to life. Heightened pressure in the pulmonary circulation drastically lowers the level of oxygen delivered to the heart—thence throughout the body—by the lungs and impairs the removal of waste materials from cells and tissues throughout the body. The result is both progressive shortness of breath, as the lungs and heart labor under increasing strain, and marked fatigue as muscles flag from lack of energy.

The condition is uncommon and occurs in five times as many women as men. It is seen more often—for unknown reasons, possibly a coincident genetic susceptibility—among those with the various rheumatic diseases. It is especially associated with the presence of anticardiolipin antibody (ACL), one of the markers of the antiphospholipid antibody syndrome (see Chapter 6), which is, in turn, one of the key diagnostic definers of lupus. Frequently, patients with pulmonary hypertension have also experienced Raynaud's phenomenon, discussed earlier in this chapter. And it can apparently be triggered by certain drugs (it was, for example, seen in the mid-1990s in association with certain appetite suppressants, since removed from the market; amphetamines and other appetite curbs have also been implicated).

Lupus patients, especially those who have other predisposing factors such as ACL and/or Raynaud's, should take active preventive measures. These are basically the same prudent precautions taken to guard against heart and circulatory disease and respiratory troubles, generally: Prevent and treat elevated blood lipids, with diet and with drugs if needed; exercise in moderation; keep chronic metabolic problems such as diabetes under firm control; and above all, *don't smoke.*

Pulmonary hypertension is differentiated from a variety of conditions with some similar symptoms by a combination of diagnostic techniques, which may include electrocardiography (ECG), echocardiography, pulmonary function testing, angiography (blood-vessel visualization), and possibly lung biopsy.

Treatment generally focuses on vasodilators—drugs designed to reduce arterial pressure by dilating the blood vessels; anticoagulants may also be used to prevent the formation of blood clots. In recent years, there has also been some promising use of intravenous prostacyclin, also known as prostaglandin I_2, one of a group of substances found naturally in various body tissues; it acts as both a vasodilator and a clot inhibitor.

Only one oral medication specifically for the treatment of pulmonary hypertension has been approved by the FDA to date. Bosentan (Tracleer) blocks the action of a natural substance, found in unusually high concentrations in the plasma and lungs of pulmonary hypertension patients, that narrows blood vessels and elevates blood pressure. It poses two major risks, however: birth defects and liver toxicity. In order to assure careful monitoring, the FDA ordered that bosentan be distributed only directly by the manufacturer, and it is not generally available through pharmacies.

At this writing, researchers have reported on two small trials of sildenafil (Viagra), a drug used for erectile dysfunction, in rapidly deteriorating patients with pulmonary hypertension who were not deemed candidates for surgery. The results seemed promising, with what the researchers called significant improvement; they cautioned, however, that further, considerably larger studies were needed.

If drug therapy proves ineffective, the recourse is lung transplantation.

KIDNEY DYSFUNCTION AND
END-STAGE RENAL DISEASE

One of the most critical threats in lupus is renal (kidney) dysfunction. About half of all lupus patients have some renal involvement, which may range from mild aberrations seen on urinalysis and signifying little to critical and even life-threatening dysfunction. Based on retrospective demographic studies, male lupus patients are at higher statistical risk of kidney involvement, as are patients (of either sex) with hypertension and those of African descent; other consistent associations have been seen with the antibodies anti-dsDNA, anti-Sm, and lupus anticoagulant.

Terms used to describe kidney troubles include *nephrosis, nephritis, glomerulonephritis*, and *nephrotic syndrome;* the last denotes a condition that also includes sharply elevated cholesterol levels and unusual fluid retention, with swelling of the legs and possibly other parts of the body. (The *-osis* suffix suggests degenerative changes, while *-itis* denotes inflammation. The various references to the organ itself derive from the Latin and Greek words for "kidney," respectively *renis* and *nephros*.) Collectively, all of these conditions are often referred to simply as *lupus nephritis*.

The most serious kind of renal assault involves continuing deposition of antigen-antibody complexes in the glomeruli, the minuscule tufts that constitute the kidney's filtering apparatus; it can eventually cause total impairment of function in that vital area. The result of this process is that waste materials, instead of being flushed from the body, remain in the circulation. Untreated, uremia—the medical term for this bloodstream pollution—would lead inevitably to increasing mental and physical deterioration and, ultimately, death.

A lupus patient's kidney function is therefore constantly monitored. A key clue to kidney health is assessment of the creatinine clearance rate. Creatine is a substance, produced by the liver, that furnishes energy for voluntary-muscle contraction. Enzyme conversion in the muscle in turn produces a waste product called creatinine, which is normally excreted in the urine. A high blood-creatinine level indicates a low clearance rate, suggesting serious kidney dysfunction.

Another assessment that may be performed is a test for blood urea nitrogen (BUN); the test determines the portion of the nitrogen in the blood derived from urea, a metabolic end-product that is another usual component of urine. Again, high levels may hint at kidney dysfunction. This test is less definitive, however, since elevated BUN may occur temporarily in conditions other than renal disease and may also be caused by certain drugs (which may either raise the levels or affect the accuracy of testing).

A third diagnostic procedure is kidney biopsy, removal of a small amount of kidney tissue for microscopic examination. Years ago, kidney biopsies were performed routinely, even when nothing in the urine suggested any trouble. That is no longer a standard practice. The procedure can be of great value in some situations—but it *is* surgery, and it need not be performed in every instance of suspected kidney dysfunction. If urinalysis shows that renal function is deteriorating, biopsy can be of great value in determining appropriate therapy. And a sudden decline in kidney function, with no warning, could signal renal vein thrombosis (clot formation), a critical condition requiring prompt intervention in the form of anticoagulants or even surgery; such a situation may require biopsy to determine the exact nature of the threat.

The drugs found most effective in treating renal involvement are the immunosuppressants (see Chapter 4), sometimes in combination with corticosteroids; the "standard" has been cyclophosphamide (Cytoxan), and the newer agent mycophenolate mofetil (CellCept) has also proved useful. These potent drugs do present significant hazards, and there is a continuing search for drugs, both immunosuppressants and others, that will be at least as effective, with fewer adverse effects.

Intravenous immunoglobulin (IVIg) has also been used experimentally to treat lupus nephritis (as well as some other lupus complications) and appears beneficial in some cases, but more extensive trials are needed.

When kidney impairment has become potentially life-threatening, and medications are ineffective—a level of impairment referred to medically as "end-stage renal disease"—there are two possible recourses.

One is hemodialysis, periodically filtering the patient's blood through a mechanical device outside the body, an "external kidney," to remove waste materials. The procedure has literally been a lifesaver for many patients, and nearly 300,000 Americans are receiving dialysis today. Overall disease activity and need for medication are likely to decrease when patients are receiving dialysis, and importantly, survival rates increase markedly. Indeed, in some patients on dialysis—a reported 30 to 40 percent—the deterioration is reversible; they may recover renal function and be able to discontinue dialysis.

The second alternative is kidney transplant, and patients who have received dialysis for a while have sometimes subsequently opted for transplant. Kidney transplant was first performed successfully in 1954, between identical twins. Within the next two decades, the surgery had become routine, due largely to two factors: (1) the development of ways to keep a kidney viable over many hours and many miles, so that it could be safely transported to a donor some distance away; (2) careful histocompatibility matching between donors and recipients, to minimize the possibility of rejection. New and improved drugs to dampen rejection reactions have also become available; they include the immunosuppressants, mentioned in Chapter 4, as well as newer agents, including sirolimus, rapamycin, and tacrolimus.

By 1977, kidney transplants had become so common that the International Human Renal Transplant Registry decided to stop keeping track of them; its final report put the world total at that time, over the preceding twenty-three years, at close to 25,000. Within a decade, the number performed annually in the United States alone was approaching 10,000.

Histocompatibility (HLA) typing and matching had steadily become more sophisticated, and it was clear that donor-recipient matching gave transplants a decided edge. But even by the mid-1980s, transplants were still organized only on a local-area basis, and so grafts from HLA-matched donors were often unavailable. A well-matched kidney might be available at a hospital halfway across the country and could be speedily airlifted to a potential recipient, if only the need were known.

In 1987, a kidney-sharing program involving transplant centers throughout the United States was begun under the auspices of the United Network for Organ Sharing (UNOS). Instead of relying on what might be available locally, the focus is now on matching, with organs quickly shipped anywhere in the United States for implant in those who are compatible with the donor's key HLA pattern. The aim of the program is maximal use of matched transplantations, for optimal survival. ("Survival" here refers only to survival of the *kidney*. When the transplanted organ fails or is rejected by the patient's immune system, it is replaced; the patient may need to be on dialysis while a second suitable kidney is located.)

In 2000, in the *New England Journal of Medicine*, UNOS summarized the results of nearly 89,000 kidney transplant operations reported to the registry during the twelve-year period from late 1987 to late 1999. The ten-year organ survival rate for the approximately 7,600 HLA-matched grafts (8.5 percent of the total) was 52 percent; that for mismatched kidneys was 37 percent—a significant difference.

Some had worried that implant delay due to shipping time might adversely affect the outcome; when local versus long-distance transport was figured into the calculations, that turned out not to be the case, and matching still won out. The report commented that only 13 percent of the HLA-matched donor-recipient pairs were from the same locality; without the sharing program, only about 2 percent of patients overall would be able to receive matching kidneys.

The report also noted that age is an apparent factor in graft survival—the age of the donor, not that of the patient receiving the transplant. Even in HLA-matched organs, the average ten-year survival rate drops to 30 percent with donors above age sixty.

With kidney transplant a truly lifesaving possibility for those with lupus nephritis—it is also considerably less costly than dialysis—it is unfortunate that so many patients are unable to benefit from it. At any given time, an estimated 45,000 people in the United States are hoping for renal transplant; only about 8,000 kidneys are available each year. (There is also a shortage of other transplantable organs, such as hearts and livers.)

Nearly 80 percent of kidneys donated for transplant come from people who have died in accidents or from other causes not affecting the health of their kidneys. The Uniform Anatomical Gift Act has made it possible for people to carry a card, with legally binding language recognized in all states, donating their organs in case of death. But fewer than 15 percent of our citizens carry donor cards; in the absence of such directives, distressed families must make organ-donation decisions at an already difficult time, and the result is often that the organ—and renewal of health to a waiting recipient—is lost.

6

APS, Pregnancy, and Problems of Both

This chapter singles out two conditions for discussion.

One is a disorder that has only relatively recently been recognized as a member of the family of autoimmune diseases, a family that includes lupus along with the more familiar rheumatoid arthritis, Raynaud's phenomenon, Sjögren's syndrome, among others. It's called the *antiphospholipid antibody syndrome*, or APS for short.

The other is not a disease at all but a normal condition that may pose out-of-the-ordinary problems for a woman who has lupus: pregnancy.

Sometimes, these two—pregnancy and APS—may interact, posing quite serious, though not necessarily insurmountable, hazards.

STATISTICAL RISKS

It has long been known that pregnancy poses special problems for many lupus patients. To begin with, many find it difficult to conceive. And if they do succeed in becoming pregnant, the outlook—statistically, at least—has not been heartening. There have been wide variations in data reported, however, and physicians now recognize that these sweeping statistics simply can't be applied across the board—or relied upon as medical care and knowledge become more sophisticated.

At one time, pregnancy seemed such a formidable—and unpredictable—threat that there was general agreement that lupus absolutely precluded childbearing, and that if conception occurred, therapeutic abortion should be performed.

That thinking has radically changed. Not all patients are at equal risk. Some are doubtless wise to avoid conceiving a child. Others, however, can probably contemplate pregnancy with few qualms (though not without sensible precautions). And the physician can now offer some guidance to help the patient make this important decision.

The general prospects of pregnancy for women with lupus are far better than they were a generation ago. Recent studies at major university hospitals in a number of countries have looked at the outcomes of pregnancies in lupus patients over the past thirty to forty years. Live births, once deemed likely in fewer than half of lupus patients, can now be expected, based on current figures, in at least two-thirds of all cases. Figures from some medical centers are now much higher; in a Johns Hopkins–University of Maryland collaborative study reported in 2003, 85 percent of pregnancies in lupus patients over a sixteen-year period resulted in live births. Prematurity is still a problem, with reported rates ranging from 20 to 35 percent, but those figures continue to fall as medical understanding and risk management improve.

Because no two women with lupus are alike, many factors come into play during pregnancy, and many questions arise: Are the perils the same throughout pregnancy? What connection might the risks have to lupus flares? Are there other conditions that might overlap and interact with lupus to pose additional problems?

Correlations of certain maternal characteristics *prior to* pregnancy with the outcomes of pregnancy have provided a great deal of information. Seriously impaired kidney function, or impaired function of any other major organ or system, is not a good omen for successful pregnancy (but a brief bout of nephritis during the pregnancy does *not* appear, by itself, to be correlated with a poor outlook). Severe flare of disease during a prior pregnancy that began in remission suggests that the same thing may occur again in future pregnancies—although other factors may have accounted for the prior episode, not excluding inappropriate or inadequate medication or another aspect of health care. A state of complete remission at the time of conception *and* for the prior six months (at least) has a better prognosis for success, while active disease at the time of conception is statistically associated with a higher incidence of complications and adverse outcomes. During the pregnancy, prompt control of potential threats—lupus flares, increases in blood pressure, faltering kidney function—appears to be the key factor.

THE ANTIPHOSPHOLIPID ANTIBODY SYNDROME

I have a new doctor, and when he took my history and found out that I'd had two miscarriages, he said he was surprised that nobody had ever tested me for the antiphospholipid antibody syndrome. He ordered the tests right away, and I was positive for anticardiolipin antibodies and for lupus anticoagulant, too. Before this, my doctors weren't sure that I had lupus, but my new rheumatologist says that with the other tests I had, this confirms it, since it's also part of the diagnosis of lupus.

Further clarification of the relationship of lupus and pregnancy has come with the recent recognition of the relevance of the family of antibodies called antiphospholipids. They are antibodies against substances found universally in the membranes of cells. Although their existence has been known for several decades, it was not until the late 1980s that the significance of APS in lupus generally, and in pregnancy in particular, began to be appreciated. The antiphospholipid antibody syndrome now ranks as a distinct autoimmune disease, and like several of the others, it has been found to "overlap" lupus with hitherto unexpected frequency. In Great Britain, the condition is sometimes termed *Hughes syndrome* after Graham R. V. Hughes, the physician who first identified it as a distinct disorder in 1983, after he and his colleagues had recognized the connection between certain co-existing antibodies and a distinctive constellation of clinical findings.

It should be emphasized that although the syndrome happens to have been first described in association with lupus, the antibodies in question are not exclusive to lupus and, until the late 1990s, played no part in diagnosing the disease. Now, evidence of APS is one of the key diagnostic criteria established for lupus by the American College of Rheumatology (ACR), as noted in Chapter 2. Although these antibodies are found in an estimated 2 to 5 percent of the general population (the proportion is a little higher in the elderly), they occur in approximately 35 percent of those with other autoimmune disorders, especially lupus or Sjögren's syndrome; the proportion appears to be even higher in youngsters with lupus, perhaps much higher (two studies, in the United States and Italy, involving lupus patients aged sixteen and under, found such antibodies in 65 percent and 80 percent, respectively). Moreover, in those with lupus, the presence of anti-phospholipids is associated with particular risks, especially—though not exclusively—in pregnancy.

One clue to the possible presence of antiphospholipids is persistent false-positive testing for syphilis, seen repeatedly over at least six months with more than one type of test. (People without lupus may also test falsely positive for syphilis, and such tests, by themselves, are not necessarily predictive of problems, in pregnancy or otherwise.)

Two specific antibodies have emerged as especially significant in lupus generally and in pregnancy in particular. Both may be detected by blood tests. Both are associated with circulatory problems and with fetal loss.

One is called anticardiolipin (ACL), and it reacts particularly with the phospholipids of cells lining blood vessels. It has been linked to a variety of unexpected incidents generally, including heart attacks and strokes in young people; phlebitis; the development of certain heart-valve abnormalities; thrombocytopenia; and, in pregnancy, recurrent miscarriages or fetal death, associated with abnormal (fetal) heart rate, after the first trimester. ("Ordinary" miscarriages, often traceable to developmental mishaps, typically take place earlier; lupus patients have a somewhat higher incidence of miscarriages in the first trimester, as well.) In some studies, the risk of fetal loss in those with this antibody has been estimated to be close to 60 percent.

Israeli researchers reported in the 1990s on an experiment in which they injected ACL antibodies from lupus patients into pregnant mice (not special mouse strains developed for research but ordinary healthy mice). The mice developed thrombocytopenia and experienced increased fetal loss. And, the researchers added, the same thing happened to mice injected with ACL from persons who did *not* have lupus—so the key factor was ACL, not lupus.

Anticardiolipin antibody has also been associated with *pulmonary hypertension*, a condition of elevated blood pressure in the pulmonary circulation. Heightened pressure in the pulmonary circulation lowers the oxygen level supplied to the heart and to all of the body's tissues, with resultant breathing difficulty and marked fatigue. Smoking may be a contributory factor, as may other conditions affecting the lungs or the heart. (See Chapter 5 for more about pulmonary hypertension.)

ACL is found, at one time or another, in about one-third to one-half of people with lupus. They often have what has been termed "atypical" lupus, which doesn't quite fit the American College of Rheumatology diagnostic criteria, and they may test negative for antinuclear antibodies (ANA).

The second significant antibody is called lupus anticoagulant (LAC); it's found in about one-tenth of lupus patients. Its name would seem to suggest that it prevents coagulation (clotting) of blood, creating a tendency to hemorrhage. Indeed, its presence is signaled by an assay (called the partial thromboplastin time, or PTT, test) that shows clotting time to be prolonged.

But the name, despite the test, is misleading: LAC is almost never associated with excessive bleeding. On the contrary, the link is with an inclination, in some people with the antibody, to form obstructive clots, or thrombi, especially in veins (venous thrombosis), sometimes associated with pulmonary emboli, fragments of these clots that lodge in the lungs. In pregnancy, LAC has been linked to miscarriage or stillbirth due to thrombi in the placenta; the loss typically takes place in mid-pregnancy.

Clinically, APS has also been associated, in significant proportions of patients, with several other disorders. They include particular neurological problems, notably, seizures or migraine headaches; joint pain and inflammation; *livedo reticularis*, patchy discoloration of the skin caused by dilation of small blood vessels; avascular necrosis of bone (even when corticosteroids, with which this condition is usually associated, are *not* being taken); leg ulcers; hemolytic anemia; and various other troubles traceable chiefly to circulatory problems, including thromboses both major and minor. All APS-related difficulties are exacerbated by smoking and by uncontrolled blood pressure, diabetes, and hyperlipidemia (high levels of cholesterol, triglyceride, and other substances in the blood).

Overall, in women who have suffered unexplained recurrent miscarriages (whether or not they have lupus), various studies have found APS in proportions ranging from 8 to 42 percent, while the reported prevalence of these antibodies in groups of obstetric patients in general has ranged from 0 to 10 percent. (ACL has been more consistently related to fetal loss than has LAC.) Clearly, there is a significant connection.

In October 1998, at a special workshop held in Sapporo, Japan, following an international conference on the subject of antiphospholipids, preliminary diagnostic criteria—often referred to among rheumatologists as the "Sapporo criteria"—were formulated for the syndrome. The criteria (which we've condensed here) include two based on clinical findings and two on laboratory assays. One of the former clearly applies only to women. The clinical measures are:

1. One or more confirmed episodes of arterial, venous, or small-vessel thrombosis.
2. At least one episode of unexplained death of a structurally normal fetus after ten weeks of pregnancy; *or* at least one episode of premature birth (before the thirty-fourth week of pregnancy) of a structurally normal fetus, due to preeclampsia, eclampsia, or severe placental insufficiency; *or* three or more unexplained consecutive spontaneous abortions (miscarriages) before the tenth week of pregnancy.

The lab-test standards are:

1. High levels of ACL antibody on two or more occasions at least six weeks apart.
2. Lupus anticoagulant found on two or more occasions at least six weeks apart by particular, specified methods.

The definite diagnosis of APS requires that at least one of the two clinical criteria, plus at least one of the two laboratory criteria, be met. That is, although the antibodies may be present, a patient cannot be said to have the syndrome unless there is also clinical evidence.

As with all of the autoimmune diseases, the cause of the antiphospho-lipid antibody syndrome is unknown but—as with all of the autoimmune diseases—there is persistent suspicion of an inborn susceptibility, with an infectious agent, possibly a virus, as the trigger.

Very little exploration as to cause has been undertaken so far. It's interesting, though, to note that in one study by a group at the More-house School of Medicine in Atlanta, reported in 2003, evidence of exposure to cytomegalovirus (CMV) was found in two-thirds of a group of patients with APS. CMV is a member of the herpesvirus family—the family to which Epstein-Barr virus (EBV), an emerging suspect in lupus itself, also belongs.

A study by a German research team, on the other hand, found an association of antiphospholipid antibodies with an entirely different virus, called parvovirus B19. This virus is most familiarly associated with a common, mild childhood infection called *erythema infectiosum* and popularly known as "fifth disease" (the reasons for that label are obscure and believed to stem from a long-ago ranking on someone's list of childhood ills characterized by rashes). The chief symptom of fifth disease is a red rash that comes and goes over a period of two to three weeks, sometimes accompanied by flu-like malaise. In adults, who are occasionally struck by it, there may also be joint pain and fever. The German investigators found evidence of prior B19 infection in more than 85 percent of their subjects, both adults and children, who were positive for antiphospholipid antibodies.

Should that test result be regarded as a condition to be treated, *in the absence of problems?* Remember that diagnosis of the *syndrome* requires not just test-tube data but clinical evidence as well. Should patient and physician wait until that evidence appears—or take preventive steps?

On the one hand, as a general rule, overmedication isn't deemed a very good idea, and that would include treating an "illness" when the patient isn't sick. On the other hand, much of medicine as practiced in the twenty-first century is *preventive*—intended to preclude the need for complex and sometimes drastic therapies. Certainly the worst potential effects of APS, such as massive thromboses or heart attacks, can be devastating.

Knowledgeable and experienced physicians generally agree that detection of these antibodies should be taken as a warning and a call for minimal preventive measures. They include avoidance, with aggressive treatment if indicated, of factors known to add to the risk: smoking, high blood pressure, high cholesterol and other lipids, uncontrolled diabetes, oral contraceptives, and unnecessary physical stressors such as cosmetic surgery.

And in the judgment of many physicians, the regimen might sensibly include one of several agents observed to have a salutary effect in preventing thrombotic events. These include aspirin, more potent prescription blood thinners such as heparin, the lipid-lowering drugs known as "statins" (which may also confer protection against osteoporosis and avascular necrosis), and hydroxychloroquine (Plaquenil), already a staple of the lupus medicine cabinet.

That threat of thrombosis is the most prominent peril in APS, since it poses a potential risk of critical organ damage if blockage of key vessels occurs. Thus, thorough evaluation, if APS is suspected, is truly vital. And because it is now recognized that there are *other* conditions (having no known connection with lupus or with APS) that can also create what doctors call a "hypercoagulable state"—that is, a state of thrombosis risk—extensive diagnostic investigation may be needed to pinpoint the exact cause(s), since preventive therapies may differ. One prominent example of such conditions is *hyperhomocystinemia,* excessive quantities of an amino acid called homocysteine; the condition may also be familial and can appear independently or may coexist with APS. That condition requires different or additional prophylactic treatment, including dietary adjustments and/or certain nutritional supplements.

PREGNANCY: PLANNING AHEAD

Now, let's take a look at the impact of lupus on pregnancy—not only the APS-associated perils but others as well.

> I have APS, and I've had blood clots that have traveled to my lungs. I'm now taking a regular blood thinner. I don't know yet if I want to try to get pregnant, since I know that a lot of women who have APS experience complications. My doctor says, though, that many women in my situation do have babies, and if my APS and my lupus stay under good control, he thinks I could, too. He says he would see that I get referred to an obstetrician who deals with a lot of high-risk pregnancies and has taken care of women with lupus and APS.

It's generally wise, if you have lupus and decide to have a baby, to view it as a high-risk undertaking. That term, in this context, doesn't mean an assumption that something will go wrong. It means that all possible precautions should be taken and that problems may nevertheless occur and should be anticipated.

Safeguards recommended for every pregnancy should be taken especially seriously, from the moment you know you want to conceive (don't wait until the pregnancy is confirmed):

- Don't drink alcohol. Period. No exceptions.
- Don't smoke. Period. No exceptions. Avoid places where other people are, or might be, smoking.
- Don't use any other "recreational" drugs—or for that matter, any medicinal substances or supplements unless they're prescribed or suggested by your doctor.

- Do eat a well-balanced diet—taking into consideration any special dietary instructions given to you by your rheumatologist or your obstetrician.
- Do follow directions for medications, including any supplements your physician may recommend (some are essential for fetal development as well as for your own health), and report any adverse or unexpected reactions promptly.
- Above all, see your rheumatologist and your obstetrician regularly, meaning as often as they have advised.

    Your obstetrician should be a specialist with extensive experience in managing high-risk pregnancies, preferably in lupus patients; should be in close touch with your rheumatologist; and should want to see you much more frequently than women with uncomplicated pregnancies, especially after the first three months—which may mean several times a week during the second trimester and even daily during the final three months.

We cannot overemphasize the importance of this continuing medical oversight: It's *vital*. Every single survey of pregnancies in lupus patients in recent years has included the observation that improved outcomes have invariably reflected three key factors:

- Early and continued optimal basic therapy for lupus to keep things on as even a keel as possible and to prevent problems.
- Careful, frequent monitoring, so that incipient threats are recognized the moment they appear, not after they have become full-fledged crises.
- Continuing control, with appropriate therapy, of such potential hazards as hypertension, the risk of thrombosis, and flares compromising kidney function.

Needless to say, all of these depend upon a close and continuous collaboration between patient and physician.

Don't even *think* about home birth, or even childbirth at a free-standing "birthing center." The latter has often proved to be an appropriate and even ideal setting for an uncomplicated, risk-free delivery under the care of an experienced nurse-midwife, but these centers are intended *only* for such deliveries.

A woman with lupus (or for that matter, any other chronic condition that poses the slightest risk to the well-being of mother or child) should plan for delivery to take place at a hospital. The hospital should be one that is equipped to care for premature or otherwise distressed infants or has ready access to such a facility—not because anything *will* go wrong, but *just in case* something does.

Because lupus has been known to flare following childbirth, it's a good idea to plan ahead for that contingency and to make arrangements for alternative or assistant child care during the immediate postpartum period.

You should also be aware of two precautions concerning pregnancy that apply to all women, with or without lupus.

The US Public Health Service recommends that all women of child-bearing age who might possibly become pregnant take 0.4 milligrams of folic acid each day. This B vitamin has been shown to help reduce the risk of neural-tube defects (NTDs), malformations of the fetal brain and/or spinal cord. The reason for taking the vitamin even if you are not pregnant is that the fetal defects can occur in the first month, before pregnancy has been confirmed.

A word is necessary, in connection with this subject, about a particular kind of testing during pregnancy. There is a substance called alpha-fetoprotein (AFP), produced mainly by the fetal liver and not found in any significant quantity in the blood of adults. A test for AFP is routinely performed on an expectant mother's blood at about the fourteenth to sixteenth week of pregnancy. Although a somewhat heightened AFP level is expected and normal, unusually high concentrations are statistically associated with (though by no means proof of) NTDs.

If high AFP levels are found, further testing is performed in an effort to find the reason. Broad surveys involving thousands of pregnancies boil down the data this way: About 40 percent of raised AFP levels are actually found to reflect NTDs; in a bit more than a quarter of the cases, other abnormal fetal conditions are present; and in about one-third, the babies are perfectly normal. Thus, high levels of AFP may signal something worrisome in about two-thirds of cases.

These figures may not hold for lupus patients, however. In one study, the Maryland state health department followed a cohort of pregnant women, both with and without lupus, performed AFP testing, and correlated those findings with pregnancy outcomes. High AFP levels were found in 7.4 percent of the lupus patients, versus only 2.6 percent of the control (non-lupus) subjects—nearly triple the rate. But the higher proportion was *not* associated with a higher incidence of babies with defects. Rather, it appeared to reflect a higher likelihood of premature birth; it was also associated with the mother's taking higher doses of prednisone.

The second warning for pregnant women in general concerns ACE (angiotensin-converting-enzyme) inhibitors, a group of drugs used to treat hypertension (high blood pressure). These agents, the FDA has warned, can cause serious or even fatal fetal damage if they're taken during the second and third trimesters (the last six months) of pregnancy. If you're taking hypertension medication and have learned that you're pregnant, you should discuss the issue with your physician and be sure that your treatment is—and will continue to be—compatible with your pregnancy. Newer alternatives to the ACE inhibitors are available.

ON THE ALERT

Throughout pregnancy, as we've stressed, monitoring must be done, with close tabs kept on both lupus activity and fetal progress. Medications may be added and subtracted to keep the disease under the best possible control, especially to treat nephritis (kidney inflammation) and other similarly serious developments.

If you've been pregnant before and you miscarried, or you have any history of blood clots, your doctor will probably want to test for those trouble-making antiphospholipid antibodies, if such testing hasn't already been done; the tests may be deemed desirable even in the absence of prior problems. Two or more tests several weeks apart may be done in order to confirm the results.

If there seems to be a definite risk of your developing clots that will threaten you and/or the fetus, special prophylactic measures may be taken. During the period of heaviest risk, in mid-pregnancy, prednisone dosage adjustments may be required. Or prevention may take the form of "blood-thinning" medication, perhaps something as simple as regular doses of ordinary aspirin, perhaps a more powerful prescription drug, such as heparin; it is, of course, vital that such a therapeutic regimen be faithfully followed.

Another critical threat is a condition called *preeclampsia*, or sometimes *toxemia of pregnancy* (a misnomer; there is no toxin involved). The complication occurs in 5 to 7 percent of all pregnancies in this country—but in about 20 percent of pregnancies in lupus patients.

Preeclampsia is signaled by a rise in blood pressure and/or proteinuria—again, one of the reasons that frequent physician visits, with pressure checks and urinalyses, are vital; preeclampsia is virtually symptomless, except that there may be some fluid retention, with swelling around fingers and ankles, and slightly greater than expected weight gain. Any of these signs and symptoms can suggest other problems, including a lupus flare, which underscores the importance of having an experienced physician carefully following the entire pregnancy.

Preeclampsia strikes in the latter months of pregnancy and is considered a major threat to both mother and baby if it progresses. Hospitalization is generally in order, with the baby delivered as quickly as possible, which may mean necessary induction of labor or cesarean section despite likely prematurity, since prematurity is the lesser threat under these circumstances. (Sometimes this complication arises extremely late in pregnancy, close to the expected delivery date.)

Of course, in addition to constant monitoring of the mother's health, the baby-to-be is closely observed, as well, to assure normal growth and development and healthy vital signs. Sonograms—ultrasound visualizations—along with heartbeat monitoring attest to fetal progress. Monitoring is especially intense after the fetus becomes viable—able to survive outside the womb—at about the twenty-fourth to twenty-sixth week of pregnancy.

Actually, as soon as fetal movement has started (most women become aware of these movements by about the eighteenth or twentieth week), the woman herself is an important monitor. As pregnancy progresses into the sixth and seventh months, most mothers-to-be develop a familiarity with their baby's characteristic movements. Any slowing or other change in these movements may mean trouble and should be reported to the doctor immediately, since speedy delivery can sometimes rescue an infant threatened by incipient failure of placental circulation.

Sometimes, deciding how to proceed when fetal distress—or potential distress—threatens can be a very close judgment call. On the one hand, removing the baby prematurely from the relative safety of the womb to the harsh environment outside cannot be contemplated lightly. But neither can continued exposure to elements in the woman's circulation that may cause harm to the child. The balance is a delicate one, and the decision must be made by an experienced physician *and* an informed patient.

MEANWHILE, ABOUT MOM'S LUPUS . . .

Although there are exceptions, in the majority of cases there is unlikely to be a worsening of lupus during pregnancy; studies have shown that exacerbations occur in only a minority of cases. Most of the complications we've mentioned seem to be due more to pregnancy than to lupus. A rash may erupt temporarily, but that's not considered serious.

More likely is a flare following childbirth. Hormonal realignments, especially the sudden drop in progesterone—the ovarian/placental hormone that has helped to sustain pregnancy—may be the possible trigger for such events. (There may also be an *apparent* spurt of postpartum hair loss. It's actually unrelated to lupus and reflects an increased growth of hair during pregnancy with a subsequent return to normal.)

In general, most medications taken regularly will be continued during pregnancy and will not harm the fetus. If steroids are needed, prednisone or prednisolone is generally preferred, since the way these drugs are metabolized in the placenta limits the amount that reaches the baby. (Some other corticosteroids cross that barrier intact and are used only if an effect on the baby is deliberately intended. One is dexamethasone, which may be given to the mother when premature birth is imminent, since it has been found to speed fetal lung maturity and help to prevent serious respiratory problems in the newborn.)

Physicians have long been leery of hydroxychloroquine (Plaquenil) and other antimalarials in pregnancy, since they do cross the placenta. A recent trial by French researchers, however, in a larger group of women than those in prior studies, suggests that hydroxychloroquine, at least, is probably safe for use during pregnancy, with the occurrence of birth defects no different in kind or number from those that might be expected in the general population. The reporting physicians did caution that the number of subjects was possibly still not high enough for firm conclusions to be reached. Bearing in mind the possibly adverse effects of the chloroquines on the eyes of patients, they also noted that complete ophthalmologic exams and tests had not been done on all of the children.

Such potent immunosuppressants as azathioprine and cyclophosphamide are generally avoided in pregnancy if possible.

One adverse effect of steroids can be osteoporosis—generally only after lengthy therapy. Pregnancy, however, poses a special risk: The fetus needs calcium for bone development, and that can cause depletion in the mother's own supply, increasing the possibility of bone problems. If the mother-to-be is taking corticosteroids, calcium supplementation may be advised. (See Chapter 7 for a full discussion of osteoporosis.)

To counter possible postpartum problems, some physicians feel that it's a good idea to increase the mother's dosage of corticosteroids about the time she goes into labor, keeping it high for several weeks thereafter and then gradually tapering it. Others disagree and feel that these drugs should be given or increased (if already being taken) only in response to disease activity and not for prophylaxis. Probably, all other things being equal, less medication, rather than more, is the better choice—but as with all other matters relating to your health, it's an individual decision, and your own physician is the one to make it.

Drug considerations in breast-feeding—medications do find their way into the nursing mother's milk, albeit in very small amounts—are similar to those in pregnancy. Both rheumatologist and pediatrician should be consulted about the safety of the specific drug(s) being taken.

Antimalarials are particularly persistent and pose some risk of eye damage to the infant, just as they do in the mother, so nursing when taking these drugs isn't a good idea. High-dose salicylate therapy can pose a risk of bleeding problems. Other NSAIDs may vary in safety, since some accumulate in the body to a greater degree than others. Although low to moderate doses of corticosteroids appear to be compatible with breast-feeding, it's probably best to limit nursing to times when maternal levels are lowest (before the morning dose and in the evening), giving formula at other times; the consensus is that breast-feeding is best avoided if high doses of steroids are being taken.

In most circumstances, breast-feeding—at least to some degree—is possible and desirable, since pediatric authorities agree that breast milk is best for the baby. Prematurity, incidentally, does not preclude providing a baby with breast milk, which can be expressed for feeding in the intensive-care nursery; if an infant is too immature to suck and must at first be nourished intravenously, milk can still be pumped and frozen for later use. (Don't thaw it by high-temperature microwaving; that has been shown to diminish its valuable infection-fighting properties.)

WILL THE BABY BE OKAY?

The greatest potential risk to the baby is the possibility of premature arrival. As noted earlier, in women with lupus, the statistics tell us that there's a higher-than-usual chance of premature childbirth.

A full-term pregnancy is defined as one that lasts from thirty-seven to forty-two weeks, so that any baby born before thirty-seven weeks is technically termed premature. In fact, a baby born after thirty-five weeks is typically fine except for not-quite-ready temperature controls, which may mean just a couple of days in an incubator.

Babies born earlier than that generally have some problems and are cared for in a neonatal intensive care unit. Those problems may vary. Treatment may include measures to deal with respiratory distress, to provide adequate nutrition when a baby cannot yet suck (intravenous feeding may be needed if the digestive system is not yet operating normally), and to cope with other aspects of immaturity. Babies weighing in at three pounds or more generally do quite well; in fact, some infants weighing not much over a pound at birth have survived and grown to be bright, healthy children.

Although lupus isn't directly inherited, and the disease isn't transmitted from mother to baby, there is nevertheless a small incidence, among babies born to lupus patients, of a lupus-related syndrome generally known, for lack of a more precise term, as "neonatal lupus." It appears to stem from antibodies that cross the placenta and is associated chiefly with anti-Ro antibodies; in fact, one very broad European study found *all* cases of the syndrome occurring in mothers with anti-Ro antibodies. About 30 to 40 percent of lupus patients, overall, have these antibodies. About 10 to 20 percent of them—that is, about 3 to 6 percent of women with lupus—will give birth to babies with neonatal lupus. (After having one such child, the chances of subsequent children with the condition are about one in four.)

Neonatal lupus, unlike "regular" lupus, is not lasting. It consists of a transient rash and transient abnormalities in blood tests (these symptoms usually disappear by six to eight months of age, sometimes well before that) and may also include a condition known as congenital heart block; in various studies, the latter has been present in half or fewer of neonatal lupus cases.

"Heart block" may sound as if the heart comes to a halt. It doesn't. The phrase is a medical term for misfiring of certain electrical signals within the heart, resulting in heartbeat irregularities, occasionally serious enough to require a pacemaker.

Studies examining specific antibodies in women with lupus who have given birth to babies with congenital heart block have found anti-Ro antibodies in 98 percent; in some studies, the figure has been 100 percent. There is also a lesser association with anti-La antibodies, which have been reported in 86 percent of the patients studied (they're found in approximately 15 percent of lupus patients overall). Investigators have also tested groups of control patients—mothers who had been diagnosed with lupus, Sjögren's syndrome, or nonspecific connective-tissue disease, and delivered babies without heart block. Among these women, anti-Ro and anti-La antibodies have been identified in, respectively, 33 percent and 15 percent.

In one study at New York University Medical Center, all of a series of mothers who delivered babies with heart block were found to have anti-Ro antibodies; 80 percent had anti-La antibodies as well—figures in line with those previously cited. Some of the women had subsequent pregnancies; 21 percent of their offspring were also born with heart block. (This research was *not* focused exclusively on lupus patients. Some of the women in the study had been diagnosed with lupus at the time of their pregnancy, others with Sjögren's syndrome; still others had neither condition.) One London clinic, in an attempt to calculate risks on the basis of antibodies, estimated that 20 percent of women with anti-Ro antibodies may deliver a baby with neonatal lupus.

In short, all mothers whose babies have heart block seem to have anti-Ro antibodies—but only a minority of women with those antibodies actually deliver babies with neonatal lupus. Might there be more than one kind of anti-Ro antibody? Apparently so. In 2002, a team of Swedish researchers found that when they tested a series of new mothers who had lupus or Sjögren's syndrome and were positive for anti-Ro and anti-La antibodies, those who had babies with congenital heart block *all* tested positive for antibodies to a subgroup called Ro 52-kd.

Still, that interesting and provocative result is just that—interesting and provocative. It's *not* the hoped-for predictive factor in congenital heart block. Indeed, the researchers reported that those very same antibodies were also found in a few mothers of perfectly healthy babies; further, sometimes different pregnancies in the same mother had different outcomes, with one baby having heart block and another being healthy. They speculated that there must be "an additional mechanism or fetal factor" involved in making the babies sick—perhaps something in the environment at one time but not at another.

What about breast-feeding? Might these antibodies reach the baby that way? In women who have anti-Ro and/or anti-La antibodies, those antibodies *are* found in their breast milk, though in lower concentrations than those in the bloodstream. Still, they do not appear to affect the baby, even when the child has arrived prematurely, and breast-feeding isn't automatically contraindicated under those circumstances. But to be on the safe side, such a baby should be carefully watched for alarm signals, including rashes, and breast-feeding should be discontinued if there's any hint of trouble.

THE QUESTION OF CONTRACEPTION

Many lupus patients, like many other women, will choose to avoid pregnancy, whether because of potential complications or because of personal choice. If you're one of them, what contraceptive method should you choose?

> I had a lot of complications during my pregnancy, including thrombophlebitis and pulmonary emboli. My doctor didn't think another pregnancy was a good idea, and I went on the Pill. Then I developed these really strange, huge red lumps on my legs. My internist didn't seem to know what to make of them and said he didn't think it was anything serious, but my gynecologist sent me to a rheumatologist. She did a bunch of tests, and now I know I have not only lupus but APS. She says the lumps are something called erythema nodosum, and she took me off the Pill right away. She doesn't advise patches or shots, either—but I really don't want to get pregnant again!

There's a clear consensus that oral contraceptives ("the Pill"), which are hormones, are best avoided by lupus patients generally and by those who have APS in particular, since they pose a heightened risk of such circulatory problems as high blood pressure, vasculitis (blood-vessel inflammation), and thrombosis.

Erythema nodosum—there is no "common" name for the condition—is one form of vasculitis, giving rise to painful reddish nodules, typically on the legs but occasionally on the arms or elsewhere on the body. It's not peculiar to people with lupus, although it does tend to strike lupus patients a little more often than others. And the Pill isn't the only cause of vasculitis; it may accompany a variety of infections ranging from strep to TB, and it may also be an adverse reaction to a number of other medications, including sulfa drugs.

Since women with lupus are already at higher-than-average risk of these circulatory problems, it doesn't make sense to raise the odds. The Pill has also been known to exacerbate lupus. For these reasons, it's best avoided, even if no circulatory complications have arisen.

What of the other forms of hormonal contraception, such as injections, patches, or levonorgestrel implants (Norplant)? At least theoretically, they pose similar risks, but opinions differ among physicians. The American College of Obstetricians and Gynecologists (ACOG) finds these alternative forms to be somewhat safer for women who should avoid the standard combination oral contraceptives containing estrogen and progestin, including those with lupus, hypertension, migraine headaches, or circulatory problems. Other physicians feel that progestin-only contraception is acceptable, while still others feel that it's best to shun *all* hormonal forms of contraception.

Intrauterine devices, IUDs, are definitely best avoided, because of the possibility of perforation, bleeding, or pelvic infection. Those risks seem, for unknown reasons, to rise in women with lupus.

The ACOG suggests that for women with any sort of medical condition that may pose a risk, "nonhormonal birth control methods may be a safe and effective contraceptive choice." Most rheumatologists would probably agree that simple physical-barrier contraceptives, such as condoms or the diaphragm or cervical cap, are the best options. Although the statistical track records of these methods are somewhat inferior to that of oral contraceptives, many knowledgeable observers have pointed out that unwanted pregnancies have often been traced to misuse (failing to follow instructions) or disuse (failing to use at all). Condoms are also the only method of contraception that protects against sexually transmitted diseases, including transmission of HIV, the AIDS virus.

Remember that corticosteroids can cause amenorrhea (absence of menstruation). If you're taking one of these drugs and you miss a period, don't instantly assume that you're pregnant.

If you are absolutely sure that you don't *ever* want to bear a child—or more children—you can consider the possibility of surgical contraception, the procedure called tubal ligation or "tube tying," which cuts off the route for eggs to find their way to the uterus. Although this surgery has been reversed in a few cases, it should be viewed as permanent.

7

Osteoporosis:
Detection, Prevention, and Remedy

*I just started seeing a new rheumatologist, since my old one re-
tired, and I can't believe what I just learned. I've had lupus for
more than twenty years, and I've been on prednisone most of
that time. I had three or four different doctors over that time, actually. Not one of them mentioned that the prednisone could
cause osteoporosis—until now, when this one brought up the
subject of having a bone density scan.*

*I did start taking a little extra calcium a few years back,
since I figured I'd be having menopause in a few years. But I
don't think I've been taking enough. I've had back pain, and
I think I lost a little height, too. Depending on what the scan
says, I think my new doctor is probably going to put me on
some medication for this.*

Among the many unfortunate side effects of corticosteroids, which are
part of most lupus patients' regimens at one time or another, is a tendency to promote osteoporosis ("porous bones"), skeletal weakening
due to loss of bone substance. This condition generally afflicts women
only after menopause, but steroids, as well as certain other factors, can

increase the risk at any age. And many people are unaware that men, too, may suffer osteoporosis—generally at a later age than women.

Osteoporotic bone is prone to easy fracture, even in the absence of outright trauma. One collaborative study at Johns Hopkins University and the University of Maryland, reported in the early 1990s, found that 6 percent of the lupus patients at the two medical centers had sustained at least one fracture since their lupus was diagnosed; one in four of them had suffered multiple fractures. Those who had had fractures were somewhat older than those who had not, were on higher steroid dosages, and were also more likely to have experienced avascular necrosis (another potential hazard, discussed in Chapter 5).

There are a number of factors, in addition to taking steroids, that increase the risk. Among women generally, statistics tell us that osteoporosis occurs more frequently among those who:

- are smokers (quitting can measurably lower the risk, even after menopause);
- are of Scandinavian descent (Caucasian women in general, as well as Asian women, are more susceptible than those of other races);
- are thin and small-boned;
- experienced any periods of amenorrhea (absence of menstruation) in their teens or twenties (not uncommon in athletes, as well as in young women with eating disorders);
- have type 1 diabetes;
- had low calcium intake when they were young;
- have had close relatives with osteoporosis.

On the basis of a study reported in late 2003, it appears that patients with inflammatory bowel disease (Crohn's disease and others) may also be at higher risk of slightly reduced bone mineral density, often referred to as *osteopenia*.

Overall, according to the National Osteoporosis Foundation, the condition is responsible for more than 1.5 million fractures in the United States each year, with vertebral and hip fractures together accounting for two-thirds of the total. Other frequent sites are wrists and ribs.

Osteoporosis is typically symptomless until a fracture occurs. The spinal fractures, incidentally, are not violent, spinal cord–threatening injuries but compression fractures of the vertebrae, usually in the upper back; they curve the spine into the sadly familiar "dowager's hump." (This disfigurement, medically termed dorsal kyphosis, is not only unsightly but hazardous to health: The postural aberration can contribute to accidental falls and, because the chest cavity is compressed, it can also contribute to pulmonary problems.)

If osteoporosis is occurring, it needs to be detected promptly. X rays alone are not totally reliable for this purpose; a more sophisticated technique called dual-photon bone densitometry is better. If you are approaching or have passed menopause; if you are taking steroids, antiseizure medications, or thyroid hormone; or if you have been diagnosed with overactive thyroid or parathyroid gland, scanning should be performed regularly, at whatever intervals your physician recommends.

Since there is no doubt about the role of corticosteroids in osteoporosis, all patients who are being or will be—or *may* be—treated with these drugs should have bone density scanning, early in therapy and preferably even before steroid therapy begins, in order to establish baseline values. It should be done regardless of age, even for those only in their twenties or thirties. Thereafter, regular scanning is vital for prompt detection of adverse changes and initiation of remedial therapy if needed.

HOW IT HAPPENS

Most people assume that once adult stature is attained, bone is more or less static. In fact, human bones continue to grow in strength and density until the mid-thirties, when peak bone mass is achieved.

Like all other tissues in the body, bone is constantly broken down (resorbed) and replaced; in bone, the process is known as remodeling.

Bone consists of a protein framework, called the osteoid matrix, in which calcium—the chief constituent of bone (as well as teeth)—is deposited. Certain cells, called osteoclasts, do the breaking-down of old bone, while other cells, called osteoblasts, are responsible for building new bone. Calcitriol (the active form of vitamin D, also known as 1,25-dihydroxycholecalciferol), the thyroid hormone calcitonin (sometimes called thyrocalcitonin), and parathyroid hormone also play important roles at various points in this cycle.

The rate of remodeling varies among individuals, and it also varies with the two types of bone, which differ in structure. Trabecular or cancellous bone, which has a lattice-like structure, is characteristic of the spine; it remodels somewhat faster than cortical, or compact, bone, which is found primarily in the long bones of the arms and legs (overall, about 80 percent of the human skeleton consists of cortical bone).

After the mid-thirties, the rate of resorption begins to exceed the rate of rebuilding. The result is a decrease in bone mass and density. Effects are slight at that point, and the decrease is very gradual, approximately 0.5 percent a year. It accelerates, however, at the time of menopause in women and during the mid-seventies in both sexes (although women are affected more by this later spurt, as well).

Bone also functions as a repository for calcium, which is not only a bone-building material. Calcium is vital to a number of other processes, including neural transmission and blood clotting. It also plays a crucial role in muscle contraction (that includes the heart as well as other muscles, both voluntary and involuntary).

A relatively constant reserve of calcium, about 1 percent of the body's total, is maintained in the bloodstream to meet these additional needs. Whenever that circulating supply drops below the demand, it's brought back up to the required level by drawing upon the bones' stores. Depletion of this store of calcium without replacement triggers the insidious process of osteoporosis.

The drop in available estrogen at menopause is associated with a speed-up of bone resorption, and the reason smokers raise their risk of osteoporosis is that smoking results in abnormally low levels of circulating estrogens. One theory of the significance of estrogen holds that

its depletion somehow upsets the balance in the numbers of osteoclasts and osteoblasts, resulting in an oversupply of the former and a
shortage of the latter. The body's ability to absorb calcium apparently
slackens after menopause, as well.

While steroids may have a direct effect on bone cells, stimulating
osteoclast activity and inhibiting osteoblasts, their major impact is on
the calcium supply, since they reduce intestinal calcium absorption.
(Heavy alcohol consumption has the same effect.) In high doses or
long-term administration, steroids are also believed to reduce the levels of circulating calcitriol.

Some risk factors, including your genetic background and nutritional disadvantages you may have experienced as a child, are beyond
your control, and the medications you must take may not offer much
choice, either. But there *are* steps you can take to improve your status
in the matter of osteoporosis risk. You can certainly avoid overindulg-
ing in alcohol. You can forgo smoking—which, as you know, you
should do in any event, for multiple health reasons. Above all, you can
make an effort to deliver adequate supplies of the essential element
your bones need.

GET MORE CALCIUM

There is no question: Calcium is *the* key to the prevention of osteoporosis. And logic dictates that the earlier the awareness of that fact,
the better. The more bone mass built up by the time of the peak
period, the greater the strength of one's bones and the greater the protection from osteoporosis.

There has been disagreement, over the years, about how much calcium most people require, and individual needs may differ. At this
writing, the National Osteoporosis Foundation recommends the following as minimum daily amounts: 1300 mg for those age eighteen or
under; 1000 mg for those aged nineteen through fifty; 1200 mg for
those over age fifty. Bear in mind that these are very general figures and
that your needs may well be different, depending on your medications,

your diet, results of your bone densitometry, and other factors. Where you fit into this scheme is best discussed with your own physician.

Research in recent years has also suggested that adequate, or even extra, calcium may be helpful to one's health in other ways, in addition to osteoporosis prevention. Several studies have shown an inverse relationship between blood pressure and calcium in hypertensive people—that is, the higher the calcium intake, the lower the pressure (an effect not seen in subjects whose blood pressure is normal in the first place). Furthermore, some investigators have suggested that increased calcium may play a protective role against cancer of the colon.

Where do you get calcium? Nutritionists agree that, in general, the best source for all nutrients is the natural one: the diet. The best dietary sources of calcium, as you doubtless know, are milk and other dairy foods—cheeses, ice cream, yogurt,[1] and so on. And the good news is that those dairy foods that are best for you otherwise are also the best sources of calcium, while such high-fat dairy products as butter, cream, and cream cheese have relatively low calcium content.

As you may not know, there are other good diet sources of calcium, too. Three ounces of canned sardines (in oil, with bones), for example, provide 370 mg of calcium. Ten dried figs will give you 270 mg. An average slice of pizza (an eighth of a 15-inch pie) offers 220 mg. Three ounces of canned salmon contain 165 mg. A packet of fortified instant oatmeal supplies 160 mg, as does a cup of tomato soup made with milk. Green leafy vegetables such as collards and kale are also rich in calcium (a medium broccoli spear, cooked and drained, has more than 200 mg), and some fruit juices, breads, and cereals are fortified with calcium. Tofu and other soybean products are good sources, as well.

It may be difficult to meet your calcium needs with diet alone, however. You can also get calcium through supplements. Such supplements are available without prescription, in several forms, both brand-named and generic, including calcium carbonate (Caltrate, Os-Cal, among others), calcium citrate (Citracal), calcium phosphate (Posture-D), and others. Research has shown that calcium citrate is particularly effective because of its high absorption levels compared with some other forms;

recent analyses have shown that calcium citrate's absorption is from 22 to 27 percent higher than that of calcium carbonate. Whatever form you choose, taking the supplement with food increases its absorption. The bottom line is that if the calcium in the calcium pills you take never reaches your bones, you may as well not be taking them. Perform a simple test: Drop a tablet of the product into some ordinary vinegar. If it doesn't dissolve within half an hour, it won't dissolve in your GI tract, either.[2]

Do be sure that your physician(s) and dentist(s) know that you take calcium supplementation, since it can clash with certain other medications. Calcium supplements may, for example, interfere with absorption of the antibiotic tetracycline.

Will extra vitamin D, by itself or along with the calcium, help? Maybe; maybe not. Vitamin D supplementation combined with calcium supplements have been found useful in preventing hip fractures in the elderly (people in their seventies and eighties and up), in whom deficiency is not uncommon. Deficiency earlier in life, though, is less likely, and tests of vitamin D supplementation in younger women have shown conflicting results. Your doctor can order a blood test to determine whether your levels of vitamin D are adequate; if they're not, either calcium supplements combined with vitamin D or the addition of separate vitamin D may be recommended.

Various other foods can interfere with your body's calcium balance, whether the calcium comes from your diet, from supplements, or both. Some foods do so by lowering the level of calcium absorption. One such group of foods are those containing chemicals called oxalates, which form an insoluble substance in combination with calcium; spinach, cabbage, chocolate, cocoa, nuts, and tea are especially high in oxalates. High quantities of dietary fat—as well as too-high quantities of otherwise good-for-you fiber—can also decrease calcium absorption.

Diets unusually high in protein, sodium (as in table salt), or caffeine (three or more cups of coffee a day, or the equivalent in tea or cola drinks) can cause depletion of the body's calcium levels by increasing excretion of the mineral.

Other supplements and drugs, besides corticosteroids, may encourage a tendency to osteoporosis. Megadoses of zinc supplements or vitamin A can decrease calcium absorption, as can some antacids containing aluminum (antacids containing calcium, though, can do double duty as calcium supplements). A variety of medications—including some sedatives, muscle relaxants, anticonvulsants, and oral drugs for diabetes—can inactivate the calcitriol needed for bone rebuilding. And certain types of diuretics (drugs that reduce fluid buildup) can deprive the body of calcium by speeding its excretion.

A precaution: If you have had kidney stones—that term covers stones anywhere in the urinary tract—it's important for you to talk with your doctor before you take any calcium supplement. There are a number of distinct types of kidney stones, and some contain calcium. People who have a tendency to form calcium-containing stones shouldn't take calcium supplements.

ALTERNATIVE/ADDITIONAL MEDICINE

If you've been taking calcium supplements, and bone density scanning nevertheless reveals a continuing problem, your physician may suggest other recourses.

One is the thyroid hormone mentioned earlier, calcitonin or thyrocalcitonin (Miacalcin). This hormone acts to slow bone loss by reducing the rate of resorption. Clinical trials suggest that it acts somewhat selectively, though—that it's very effective in decreasing spinal bone loss and preventing vertebral fractures, less so in preventing bone loss in arms and legs.

Until a decade ago, calcitonin was available only in injectable form; the injection is subcutaneous—just under the skin—on an every-day or every-other-day basis. The hormone is now also marketed in intranasal (nose spray) form. It cannot be taken orally.

The calcitonin used in this country, derived from salmon, can cause allergic reactions in some people. If your physician believes the hormone may be helpful for you, skin tests may be advisable before treatment is begun, especially if you have a history of allergies—as many lupus patients do. It should also be noted that some people become "resistant" to its benefits because they produce antibodies against it, although this is less likely to occur with the intranasal form.

A class of oral drugs called *bisphosphonates* also decreases bone resorption, specifically by inhibiting osteoclast activity; they include alendronate (Fosamax), risedronate (Actonel), and others. These drugs have been found to be effective in increasing bone mass, but certain precautions must be followed in order to compensate for the fact that they are poorly absorbed: they must be taken first thing in the morning after fasting overnight and at least half an hour before anything is eaten. Unfortunately, there are a number of gastrointestinal side effects, which some people find intolerable.

A totally different approach with this class of drugs is under study. In 2002, a multinational trial, led by investigators at the University of Auckland, in New Zealand, reported promising results with a new, powerful bisphosphonate, zoledronate. Bypassing the troublesome gastrointestinal route, the drug is injected—as infrequently as once a year (intervals of three and six months were also included in the study). That initial trial, which involved only 350 women, demonstrated definite improvement in bone mineral density. Further trials, seeking evidence of fracture prevention, are now underway in much larger groups of subjects, both men and women; they are expected to take several years.

Another kind of drug, called a *selective estrogen receptor modulator* ("SERM"), was introduced in the late 1990s. Raloxifene (Evista) is a "cousin" of tamoxifen, a drug used to treat some forms of breast cancer. Taken orally, it seems to have paradoxical effects, thus far both positive: Research reports indicate that it has estrogen-like impact on spinal and hip (but not other) bone, increasing bone density, and it has anti-estrogen effects in that it may decrease the risk of estrogen-dependent breast cancer. The drug's long-term performance is being further explored to see if it may play a role in preventing heart disease or stroke, risks that some studies imply may be increased by hormone replacement therapy.

Still another sort of drug was approved by the Food and Drug Administration in late 2002 specifically for the treatment of women who are past menopause, are suffering from osteoporosis, and are considered to be at high risk for fractures. Teriparatide (Forteo), a parathyroid hormone fraction, stimulates bone formation; it must be taken by daily injection. The drug is very new, and experience with it is limited. Because a heightened risk of bone cancer emerged in animal experiments (though not in human trials), the FDA has cautioned that teriparatide must not be used for children or adolescents or for women who are pregnant or nursing; nor should it be used by anyone who has had bone cancer (or other cancer that has spread to bone) or other bone disease. Nor, generally, has the safety of the drug in prolonged use yet been established.

This sort of drug, by the way, is not intended to be added to another drug regimen, such as a bisphosphonate. It did occur to researchers that if each drug is good, together they might be even better. That has proved not to be so. In fact, two studies testing that theory were reported in the fall of 2003—one, in women, by a collaboration of researchers in five states; the other, in men, by a team at Massachusetts General Hospital. Both studies, in which some subjects were given alendronate, some parathyroid hormone, and some both, reached the same conclusion: Not only was there was no evidence of synergistic (enhanced) effect, but the alendronate appeared to *diminish* the helpful effects of the hormone.

How about fluoride? Since it is a highly effective strengthener of teeth—defending them against decay caused by bacteria-produced acids—might it have a similarly beneficial impact on bone? That thought has indeed occurred to researchers in this area, but studies have not been promising. In clinical trials in post-menopausal women, fluoride did appear to increase bone density—and also, perversely, the number of new fractures; the treatment seemed to create new bone that was dense but structurally abnormal.

Early in 2004, results of a three-year international study led by French rheumatologists, testing yet another drug, were reported. The new oral medication, strontium ranelate, appeared in that clinical trial to reduce the risk of vertebral fracture (in women who already had osteoporosis) by half, with apparent safety. Comparison was with a placebo (an inert substance); the new drug has yet to be tested directly against the agents already in use.

And if you already take a cholesterol-lowering drug, you'll be pleased to learn that several studies have shown that there appears to be an unexpected "side effect." The drugs popularly known as "statins" appear to bestow a marked lowering of the risk of hip fracture caused by reduced bone mass.

HOW ABOUT HRT?

Since a loss of estrogen raises the risk of osteoporosis in women after menopause, a crucial question for women is that of estrogen replacement therapy—ERT or, as it's more commonly called, H(for "hormone")RT (the estrogen is often coupled with the hormone progesterone to minimize the small but real risk of endometrial cancer that may be raised by estrogen alone—unless, of course, the patient has had a hysterectomy).

Postmenopause HRT has been advocated as valuable for a number of reasons over the years (aside from necessary replacement when the ovaries have been removed due to disease): relief of a variety of temporary discomforts accompanying menopause; prevention of heart and circulatory problems that seem to occur more frequently in older women (estrogen appears to have a favorable effect on cholesterol ratios); and as one protection, along with calcium and other measures, against osteoporotic fractures.

But is it safe? Or do the risks outweigh the benefits? The question has been hotly and widely debated, in both the medical journals and the public media, over the past few years; we'll try to sum up the essentials rather than rehash the entire controversy here.

A decade ago, across-the-board HRT was endorsed virtually unanimously by policy-setting medical groups both in and out of government. Now, some of those experts have expressed doubts.

Positions may change radically in medicine, with time and new (or newly recognized) information, and the changing position on HRT is a prime example of this. At a 2002 conference sponsored by the Office of Research on Women's Health at the National Institutes of Health, some who had previously hailed HRT's role in preventing heart disease flatly recanted, observing that in many cases in one large study, there had been confounding factors. That study had followed a large number of women using *various forms* of HRT as well as others who hadn't had the replacement therapy; the research had seemed to show far better health in the users on all counts. Closer scrutiny revealed that many women who had chosen HRT and remained healthier turned out to be the sort of people who also took *other* health-promoting measures: They ate more healthful diets, they paid careful attention to their doctors' orders, and so on.

Part of the problem lies in the definition of the substances being investigated. The term "HRT" does not denote a single substance, although some headlines and broadcast news reports have made it seem so. The estrogen may take the form of one of the natural human estrogens, estradiol or estrone. More commonly, the estrogen is formulated as *conjugated equine estrogens* (yes, from horses—specifically, pregnant mares), which the body converts to human forms. It may come in various dosages. It may or may not be combined with another hormone, progesterone, which is also available in various forms (one synthetic form is usually referred to as progestin) and in various dosages.

A second study, the Women's Health Initiative trial, received even more publicity and generated major confusion in mid-2002. It focused on a product called Prempro, a combination of 0.625 mg conjugated equine estrogens with 2.5 mg medroxyprogesterone acetate. Its conclusion, which became something far more alarming in many newspaper headlines, was the following: "This regimen should not be initiated or continued for primary prevention of coronary heart disease." (The quotation is from the *Journal of the American Medical Association*, July 17, 2002.)

These two studies have been the largest conducted to date. The first was not controlled; subjects used a wide variety of HRT regimens. The second focused on a specific formulation of hormones. There have also been other, smaller studies. Have they agreed on anything? In fact, they have:

- *Risks.* HRT may encourage, rather than stave off, both coronary heart disease and stroke, possibly by raising lipid (especially triglyceride) levels. It may lead to gallbladder inflammation. It may raise the risk of breast cancer (possibly, some investigators believe, due to the progestin component in combination regimens). And the highest risk of all, on which all reports are in agreement, is that of blood-clot formation, pulmonary embolus in particular; that risk rises markedly.
- *Benefits.* HRT appears to reduce the risk of colorectal cancer. And it does, without question, help to prevent osteoporotic fractures.

Now, the questions:

- Might other forms of estrogen, or of progesterone, pose different benefits and risks?
- What is the relative role of the two components, in combination regimens, in the various risks and benefits?
- Might lower doses of either or both offer similar benefits with lower risks? In June 2003, the FDA approved a lower-dosage form of Prempro: 0.45 mg of estrogen and 1.5 mg of progesterone.

  In August 2003, researchers at the University of Connecticut reported the results of a four-year study of healthy postmenopausal women, testing the potential of ultra-low-dose (0.25 mg) estradiol to promote bone density. The study was controlled and double-blind (neither patients nor researchers knew until the study ended which subjects had received the test drug and which an inert placebo); short courses of progesterone were given to all of the women at six-month intervals. Result: The hormone reduced bone breakdown and raised bone density "significantly," and there were no serious side effects.
- What effect might varying delivery methods have? Estrogen can be taken by mouth, as it has been in the major studies. It can also be delivered transdermally, by skin patch; by vaginal cream; or by the most recently introduced method, a vaginal ring (Femring) that stays in place for three months, approved by the FDA

in the spring of 2003. The ring releases the form of estrogen called estradiol.

A report from French researchers in late 2003 suggested that the patch may offer significant protection. The short (six-month) trial compared groups of women wearing the patch or receiving oral estrogen and found that the patch group developed markedly lower levels of blood factors signaling a risk of thrombosis.

One precautionary tale for those considering a patch. Two Australian neurologists were confronted with an aerobics buff— she'd been pursuing the activity for years—who had recently begun suffering severe headaches, lasting several hours, following her exercise classes. She feared a brain tumor or other dire condition, but tests showed nothing of the sort. Questioning revealed that the patient had recently switched from oral to transdermal estrogen replacement—that is, via a skin patch. Intense exercise, the physicians concluded, led to vasodilation, which increased through-the-skin estrogen absorption, raising the blood level suddenly, which in turn precipitated a headache. The doctors' advice: Don't wear the patch during exercise classes. It worked.

- The bottom-line question: What does all this mean for the concerned female lupus patient who may be doubly at risk for osteoporosis, approaching menopause and also relying on prednisone or other corticosteroids to keep lupus in check?

Certainly HRT—with the possible, not yet proved, exception of the skin patch—is not advisable for a patient already at clear risk of blood clots. A five-year Danish study of some 13,000 women, reported in late 2003, also made it clear that for women with hypertension, HRT may double the risk of stroke.

Further, a Swedish study reported early in 2004 in the British medical journal *The Lancet* found that among women who had previously had breast cancer, HRT appeared to pose a definite risk of recurrence. Originally projected as a five-year comparison of HRT with other menopause-related treatment, the research was brought to an early halt because the risk to women with a history of breast cancer was deemed unacceptably high. The American Cancer Society concurred, terming use of HRT by such women "unwise."

For those not in these categories—especially if the patient is a thin, blond former athlete (that is, if she has other characteristics predisposing her to osteoporosis)—the benefits may often outweigh the risks.

In short: The decision, like many in medicine, is a highly individual one and should be made by patient and physician after careful consideration of risks and benefits.

THE BENEFITS OF EXERCISE

Finally, there is one anti-osteoporosis regimen that can be recommended without reservation: regular exercise—particularly weight-bearing exercise. Whatever other preventive steps are taken, the addition of regular exercise will without question be helpful.

Quite a few studies have definitely demonstrated the direct relationship between exercise and bone mass—and bone mass, we know, is the main factor in reducing the potential for fracture-fostering osteoporosis. Although the nature of this association isn't fully understood, it appears that in the course of exercise, the muscle activity exerts a kinetic effect on the bone to which it's attached, an effect that stimulates osteoblastic activity—that is, the formation of new bone. Conversely, it's been observed that in periods of enforced immobility—for example, when long bed rest has been necessary—a rise in the rate of bone resorption takes place, evidently due to increased osteoclast activity.

Indeed, a recent discovery hints that this factor may play a significant role in the history of osteoporosis. Many observers have noticed an increase in osteoporotic fractures over the years, an increase that's age-specific (so not attributable to the use of corticosteroids) but not accounted for by the fact that people live longer these days. Perhaps there's another reason.

A London church restoration undertaken in the 1990s required digging up the remains of parishioners buried during the eighteenth and early nineteenth centuries. Their ages at the time of death were all known. When scientists, curious about changes over time, scanned the femurs (thighbones) of female skeletons from the churchyard and compared them with those of present-day women of comparable age, they found distinct differences in rate of bone loss. It was much higher in the modern women, even prior to menopause (in fact, in the exhumed bones, there had been *no* significant premenopausal loss).

The investigators' report, noting that the difference could be due to many factors, nevertheless remarked that the women of that area, called Spitalfields, were known to have done a great deal of walking and to have worked up to fourteen to sixteen hours a day at the main local occupation, silk-weaving (in addition to caring for their children). One factor in accounting for the difference, the researchers concluded, could be a modern decrease in physical activity.

In any event, we know that loss of muscle strength, which occurs mainly through inactivity, contributes directly to loss of bone strength. Improve muscle strength, through exercise, and you improve bone strength, as well.

Weight-bearing exercise, especially, also called "skeletal loading," leads to increased muscular strength. That term refers not only to literally lifting weights but to any activity in which weight is lifted or carried, including knee bends, stair-climbing, dancing, and just plain walking. Much "aerobic" exercise promoted for cardiovascular and overall health qualifies in this area as well—except that swimming, which is by and large a splendid form of exercise, is not helpful for this purpose, since it expressly relieves weight-bearing stress. Generally, a program of moderate exercise that addresses both concerns, and provides activity for all the skeletal muscles, is the best choice for everyone. The ideal exercise fitting that description happens to be the most readily available for most people and requires no equipment at all.

The American Academy of Orthopaedic Surgeons (AAOS) strongly recommends walking as a basic daily activity in a program to prevent osteoporosis, noting that in addition to strengthening leg muscles, it peps up circulation. Start with a short walk, such as a quarter of a mile or about five city blocks, increasing the distance gradually over a period of weeks, until a routine one mile a day is reached. The academy cautions that overexertion should be avoided, and that if any discomfort or breathlessness occurs, medical consultation is in order. Walkers should also heed local air pollution alerts, since outdoor physical exertion under those circumstances can be hazardous to your health; do your strolling indoors on those days.

On the pages that follow is a simple exercise program adapted from one developed by the President's Council on Physical Fitness and recommended by the AAOS. Designed originally as a beginning program for people over age sixty, it can serve as a good start for anyone unaccustomed to strenuous activity. The "level 1" routines are the easiest, and you should feel comfortable with them, and be able to accomplish them all without difficulty, before you add the "level 2" exercises (from that point on, perform all ten at each exercise session). Similarly, try the more challenging "level 3" exercises only after you've mastered those at the previous level; then, do all fourteen each day.

Three precautions, before you begin:

1. If you've had any arthritis, other joint problem, or fracture, or if scanning has shown that you have any degree of osteoporosis, get your physician's approval first. Especially if you have suffered any injury, rehabilitative physical therapy may be recommended before you undertake any new physical activity.
2. Pay no attention to the "no pain, no gain" adage. Slight soreness, which may persist overnight—or even appear the next day rather than immediately—is not unusual when a previously inactive muscle is exercised. *Pain* is something different. It is a message from your body that something is amiss, a signal to stop what you are doing and check with your doctor.

3. If you develop any new symptoms, or if any aspect of your lupus worsens, stop the program *and* make a date with your physician. The problem may or may not be related to the exercise. If it is, it's important to clarify the connection. If it isn't, you need to find out what *is* causing it.

NOTES

1. Some people are lactose-intolerant, meaning that they can't digest milk sugar and suffer serious stomach upsets from most dairy foods. Yogurt may be a feasible alternative. Lactase tablets, containing the digestive enzyme that lactose-intolerant persons lack, are also available.

2. Also beware of products deceptively containing the word "calcium" that are not actually effective calcium supplements at all—or good for anything else, either. In 2003, the Federal Trade Commission (FTC) and the Food and Drug Administration (FDA) took action against marketers of a nostrum called "Coral Calcium," claimed falsely not only to furnish high levels of calcium but to be an effective treatment for ills ranging from cancer and heart disease to multiple sclerosis and, yes, lupus. The product was extensively promoted on various Web sites and television channels. "Seen on TV" is not a warrant of respectability. *No* supplements should be taken except after consultation with your physician.

Level 1

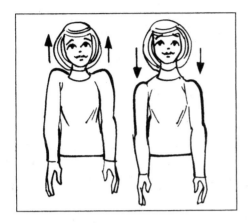

1A: Start with this simple shrug, repeating it ten times. Important: Stand straight, keep your head perfectly erect, and be careful not to lift one shoulder higher than the other (stand in front of a mirror to make sure).

Illustrations by Bill Kresse

1B: Choose a straight chair, and slide forward until you're sitting on the edge of the seat. Lift one leg, from the hip, until it's straight out, parallel to the floor. Hold it there for a slow count of three (later, if this seems too easy, you can increase the count to five or more), then lower it, as slowly as you can, to rest your foot on the floor. Do the same with the other leg. Repeat the full routine five times to start; later, increase to ten or fifteen times. Be sure to protect your lower back from strain by consciously using your abdominal muscles (this precaution is important with routines 1E and 1F as well).

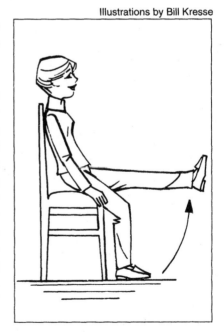

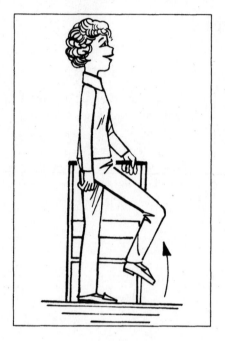

1C: Hold on to a chair back, porch railing, counter, or other convenient support and, standing perfectly straight, raise one knee as high as you can, hold for a slow count of three, and lower. Do this a total of five times (later, you can increase to ten), then repeat with the other leg.

1D: Sit in a straight chair again, but this time, sit up straight, with your back against the back of the chair, your knees bent; your feet should rest comfortably on the floor. This exercise is like 1B, except that your leg moves only from the knee down, coming up to form a straight line with your thigh.

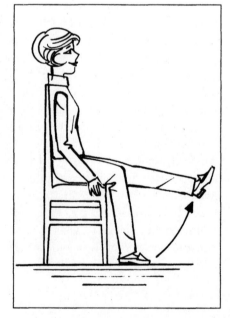

1E: Holding on to a chair or other support with both hands, raise one leg behind you, as high as you can. Important: Keep the leg straight (you should feel the pull through your buttocks, not the back of your knee), and stand erect, shoulders back and head up; don't tilt forward. Do ten times with each leg; you can do ten raises with one leg and then ten with the other, or alternate legs, as you like.

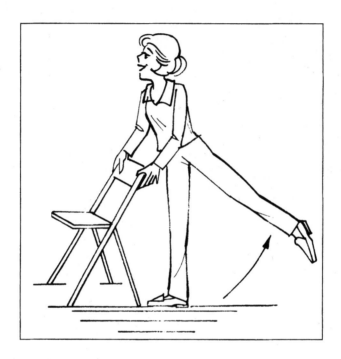

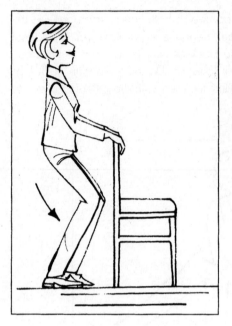

1F: Stand erect, again holding on to a support with both hands. Keeping your heels on the floor and your torso erect, bend your knees to approach a "sitting" position; go as far as possible. Return to standing position as slowly as you can. Perform this exercise ten times.

Level 2

2A: Two- to three-pound weights are suggested for this exercise; you can use household objects, such as cans of food, but weights are standardized and a great deal easier to grip firmly, so they won't slip out of your grasp. Stand erect and hold the weights at your sides, either palms forward (as shown) or palms toward your body as if holding a briefcase, whichever's more comfortable. Bend your arms to curl the weights upward; if you've begun in the second described position, allow your wrists to turn on the way up, palms toward you. Repeat ten to fifteen times, increasing later to twenty or more.

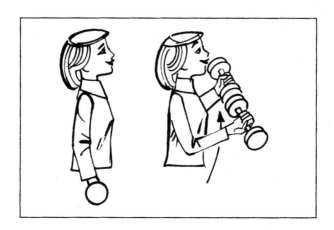

2B: Start by kneeling as shown, hands placed at shoulder width but slightly forward, arms straight. Slowly bend your arms to lower your upper body until your nose touches the floor. Important: Don't let your forearms rest on the floor. Return to the starting position by straightening your arms to lift your torso. Repeat ten times or more.

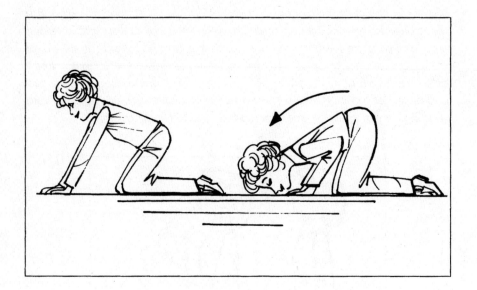

2C: Lie on one side as shown, perfectly straight, tilting neither forward nor back. Slowly raise the upper leg, keeping it straight and aligned with your body (i.e., neither forward nor backward but toward the ceiling); it may be helpful to have someone else tell you if you're performing this one correctly. Repeat at least ten times, then turn over to the other side and do the same with the other leg.

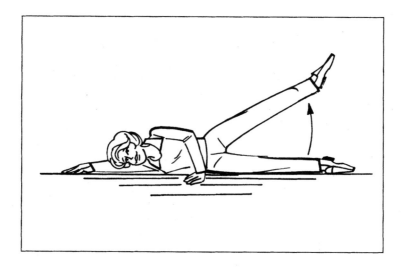

2D: Start this routine by standing with feet very slightly apart, hands on hips. Slide one leg forward, bending that knee as far as you can, at the same time swinging your arms straight forward; the heel of the other leg must remain on the floor, and the back leg and the upper part of your body should form a straight line. Perform five times with each leg, later increasing to ten.

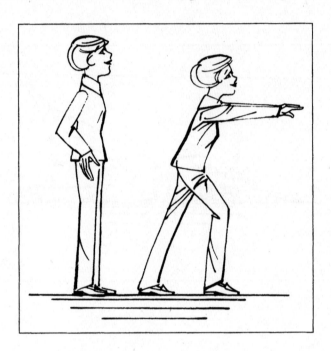

Level 3

3A: These arm curls use heavier weights— five-pounders are suggested to start—and, since simultaneous lifting (at least at first) is likely to throw off posture and balance, alternate lifts are used: Bring one weight up to your shoulder; then, as you lower that one to your side, raise the other one, continuing to alternate until you've performed the full routine at least ten times with each arm. When you feel more confident, you can try simultaneous lifting.

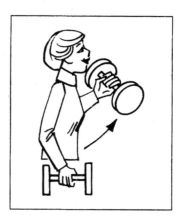

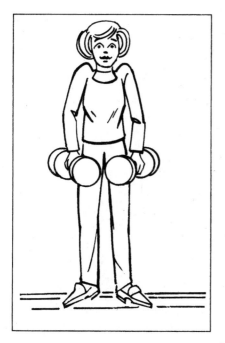

3B: This is the same as 1A, except that now you're lifting weights as you shrug your shoulders. Start with five-pound weights; try eight-pounders later, if you feel up to it.

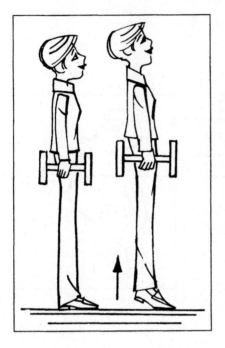

3C: For this routine, stand straight, a five-pound weight in each hand, feet shoulder width apart. Slowly rise up on your toes as high as you can, and hold as long as you can do so without losing your balance. Slowly lower your heels to the floor. Repeat ten times. Variation: Try performing with your toes turned slightly outward, like a ballet dancer (rotate your leg from the hip).

3D: Start as you did for the last exercise, standing straight, weights in your hands, feet about shoulder width apart. Slowly bend your knees—keeping your heels on the floor—as far as you can while maintaining your balance and keeping your torso erect. Then, as slowly as you can, straighten your legs to return to standing position. Repeat ten times.

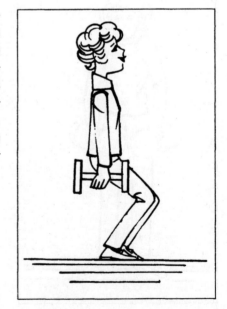

CHAPTER

8

Other Medical Questions

Chapter 5 discusses a number of conditions that, while not precisely part of lupus, are closely connected with it—as overlapping autoimmune disorders, as direct results of lupus or its treatment. Two health controversies that may particularly worry women—estrogen replacement therapy and the possible perils of breast implants—are discussed in Chapters 7 and 12. In this chapter, some additional questions and concerns—matters by no means peculiar to lupus but likely to be of special interest to many, if not most, lupus patients of both sexes.

HEART AND CIRCULATORY HEALTH

As everyone who has access to any medium of communication is aware, coronary heart disease (CHD)—damage to the heart caused by blockage of one or more of the several arteries delivering fresh blood, pumped by the heart, to the heart itself—is one of the most widespread ills on the planet. And study after study has found that lupus patients are among those in the very greatest peril. Major investigations reported in *Arthritis & Rheumatism*, the journal of the American College of Rheumatology, have pegged the relative risk of CHD in lupus patients as five to seven times the risk among the general population.

147

The potential danger (to lupus patients and others alike) is generally assessed in terms of *risk factors*—elements that, taken alone, tilt
the odds and that combine synergistically to heighten the hazards to
an alarming degree.

As you doubtless know, one factor in that life-threatening obstruction of the coronary arteries is the fatty substance called cholesterol—
actually, just one of several substances collectively known as *lipoproteins*
or *lipids*; another well-known lipid group is the triglycerides. The process is known as *atherosclerosis* (from two Greek roots referring to the
deposit of fatty material plus the hardening and diminished flexibility
of vessel walls).

Both total lipid levels in the blood and comparative levels of two
subtypes are important in predicting the risk of heart disease, and the
subtypes have emerged as perhaps even more significant. The two subtypes are HDL (high-density lipids), a higher ratio of which appears to
be protective, and the LDL—and, worse, VLDL—types (for "low" and
"very low" density), higher relative levels of which raise the risk.

Although atherosclerosis is a threat to us all, persons with lupus are
especially likely—especially during periods of active disease—to display
high lipid levels and to have notably low levels of HDL, tilting the ratio
in the "wrong" direction; lupus is also associated with higher-than-
usual levels of triglycerides. The reason isn't completely clear, but the
general inflammation that characterizes lupus probably plays a part in
narrowing the arteries and encouraging the deposit of fats; indeed,
some recent research suggests that lipids themselves can apparently
promote inflammation by provoking the immune system to launch an
artery-damaging attack. (That phenomenon isn't peculiar to people
with lupus.) Even HDL, the "good" lipids, seem to be capable of this
activity—so that people who haven't received lipid-lowering therapy
because of a perceived beneficial HDL-LDL ratio perhaps *should* be
treated if their overall levels are nonetheless high.

Additional risk-raising factors include anything else that may stress
the heart or circulatory system and is uncontrolled or inadequately
treated: hypertension, diabetes, obesity, irregularities of heart rhythm,

inflammation of the outer layer of tissue enclosing the heart muscle (pericarditis, relatively common in lupus) or of the heart muscle itself (myocarditis). Unfortunately, some of these threats can be fostered by lupus therapy, especially corticosteroids, which are associated with raised lipid levels. Lupus itself is also associated with increased blood pressure (which may be caused by kidney disease as well as by steroids). The atherosclerotic process is accelerated in some lupus patients due to circulation of certain elements called *endothelium-stimulating cells,* which seem to further encourage thickening of blood-vessel walls.

And it is now clear from several studies—notably, one conducted by physicians at New York's Hospital for Special Surgery and reported in late 2003 in the *New England Journal of Medicine*—that a major risk factor for CHD is lupus itself.

While the male sex and advanced age are generally listed as CHD risks—that is, being female and relatively young are generally protective—lupus patients should *not* count on such assumptions. And— you've heard it before, but it needs to be said again—repeated studies have demonstrated that smoking is a major factor in coronary heart disease; that effect appears to be particularly devastating in lupus.

Moreover, all factors that raise the risk of coronary heart disease or may have any ill effect on heart health or circulation generally *also* raise the risk of stroke.

Risk factors for any disease, it should be understood, are not personal predictors; their presence doesn't augur certain illness, nor does their absence guarantee good health. Rather, they are statistical reflections of *probability* based on the known traits of those who have had a particular condition. Although it's theoretically possible for coronary heart disease to occur with a total absence of risk factors, you wouldn't want to bet on it. Making every effort to lower risk factors makes sense. Prudent measures include the following:

- If you smoke, quit. If others in your home smoke, insist that *they* quit. Secondhand smoke (air-quality experts call it environmental tobacco smoke, or ETS), whatever reassurance some may offer, *is* harmful; as long as you're breathing it, it can hurt you, no matter who's holding the cigarette.

- Eat sensibly. It's possible to enjoy food and still avoid high doses of salt, sweets, and fats. Try exploring the interesting world of herbs and other seasonings. Read labels.
- If you're obese or just overweight, make every effort to lose weight. Eat less. Move around more. Try joining a program with others who share that goal; mutual encouragement helps.[1]
- If your physician has prescribed medication to lower blood lipids, follow the regimen faithfully; if you react poorly to one drug, there are others. As with the NSAIDs, there are a large and growing number of such drugs, mainly because some patients will respond better to one than to another. They're often referred to broadly as "statins" because many (though by no means all) of their generic names end with those syllables—for example, atorvastatin (Lipitor), prevastatin (Pravachol), lovastatin (Mevacor), simvastatin (Zocor), among others. Interestingly, these drugs deliver a bonus benefit: They also seem to help to diminish the risk of avascular necrosis (see Chapter 5).

Two warnings, if you're taking a lipid-lowering drug: (1) Your physician should be routinely monitoring kidney and liver function; problems, though rare, are possible and could be serious. (2) Never exceed the prescribed dosage (a precaution that applies to *any* medication); an overdose with some of this class of drugs can occasionally cause muscle damage, and your physician will also want to monitor your level of creatine phosphokinase (CPK), an enzyme reflecting such damage. If you think you may have missed a dose, don't try to make up for it; skipping a dose is safer. Call your physician promptly if you experience any persistent muscle pain or weakness.

Similarly, follow doctor's orders for treatment designed to decrease blood pressure, control diabetes, and deal with any other risk factors—and, again, let your doctor know about any unusual symptoms; they may reflect either the condition itself or an adverse effect of the treatment.

COLD SORES AND CANKER SORES

I keep having bouts of cold sores, much more often than anybody else I know. My doctor says it's sort of connected with having lupus.

I get ulcers in my mouth, it seems like at least three or four times a year. But they don't last too long, and rinsing with salt water two or three times a day seems to help. They're really not so bad compared with some of the other things that go with lupus.

Many lupus patients suffer from sometimes unsightly, sometimes painful, sometimes merely mildly uncomfortable sores from time to time, typically cold sores (around the lips) or canker sores (ulcer-like sores within the mouth). No firm statistics exist, but these sores are probably more prevalent among lupus patients—and for the same reason that lupus patients are prone to suffer from recurrent shingles: corticosteroids and other immunosuppressive therapies.

Cold sores, also popularly known as "fever blisters"—although there is no connection with either colds or fevers—are in fact caused by a virus from the very same family as the shingles virus, the herpesviruses—which, once acquired, habitually linger in the body and reemerge when resistance falters. Here, the culprit is herpes simplex virus type 1 (HSV 1), also known as HHV 1 (for human herpesvirus); most of us acquire it in childhood. Many canker sores—medically called *aphthous stomatitis*, which translates to "ulcerative mouth inflammation"—stem from the same virus, although there are also other causes. There is no cure for these bothersome lesions; the idea is to lessen discomfort while they heal at their own pace, which is usually within two weeks (you should consult your physician if such sores persist longer).

For canker sores, your physician or dentist can prescribe a mouthwash to be compounded by your pharmacist (one that many patients have found helpful combines 500 mg of hydrocortisone with 6000 units of nystatin, 250 cc tetracycline syrup, and 500 cc benadryl syrup; be very sure that this compound isn't swallowed, since it could have unintended systemic effects). Another that may be similarly prescribed is composed of equal parts benadryl, lidocaine, and the antacid Maalox. There is also a prescription drug in paste form, called amlexanox (Aphthasol), which is said to soothe and to hasten healing. Homemade solutions can also offer relief; these may include application of ice or cold compresses, salt or baking-soda pastes, and warm salt-water or baking-soda rinses.

Among nonprescription products many patients have found helpful are doconasol (Abreva) for cold sores and topical anesthetic/analgesic gels containing various strengths of benzocaine, ranging from 5 to 20 percent, for both types of lesions; the latter include Anbesol, Orabase, Orajel, SensoGard, and others. *Caution:* Don't use one of the benzocaine products if you've ever had an allergic reaction to a caine-type anesthetic (the novocaine used in dentistry, for example).

Similar ulcers may occur, less commonly, in the vagina. Your doctor can suggest or prescribe an appropriate remedy for discomfort. Over-the-counter products that have *not* been thus recommended are best avoided.

PERSISTENT ACHES AND PAINS

Sometimes the joint pain can get really, really fierce. I remember one time—it was on a weekend, of course—and no kind of analgesic I had in the house was working. I wound up stretched out on the bed, literally in tears, it was that bad, with my husband putting ice packs on every joint.

Between the lupus and the fibromyalgia, the constant pain was making me crazy. I think it's mostly the fibro, since the pain's

mainly in the muscles and tendons rather than right in the joints. I was having headaches on top of everything else, I think mostly from stress. My rheumatologist said, "I'm going to send you to a pain management clinic, because the next thing I'd have to do is prescribe opiates, and I don't want to do that." I didn't want him to, either.

Well, the pain clinic was fantastic. They really know what they're doing. I had several sessions with a physical therapist, who had other fibro patients and knew exactly where the pain was, and there was also a psychologist who told me about tricks to relax muscles and nerves. The PT sent me home with a bunch of great exercises for the trouble spots, and I also learned about TENS; the PTs all use them, and I've now got my own unit—which is not only terrific for the fibro but also works on neck tension, which helps with the headaches.

They have a doctor in charge, and he gave me a new prescription for pain, but I haven't needed it very much—and I don't even have the headaches anymore—well, maybe one every few weeks. But I used to have them every two days!

❧

Now, on top of everything else, I've started having terrible headaches. My regular doctor thinks it's migraine, and he prescribed a drug that's supposed to help—and I guess it did, some. He says there are also other drugs I could try. But he wants me to see a neurologist.

❧

I got shingles—not once, but twice; a lot of lupus patients do, my doctor says. Then, after the second time, the pain stayed on. Well, the shingles itself wasn't really painful, compared to what I had afterward. It was awful, so bad that I couldn't even sleep. And the usual pain drugs didn't work. Then my doctor

prescribed Neurontin—which isn't actually a pain pill but a
drug for epileptic seizures, only it also works on this pain,
which is some kind of neuralgia, which means it's actually in
a nerve.

Lupus is a decidedly uncomfortable disease. Sometimes, for some patients, sheer pain is a part of it—occasionally, severe, intractable pain. And sometimes there's no cure, no way to banish the cause itself. Coping is aimed at relief, and that may involve both the intensity of the pain itself and the patient's perception of and reaction to it, a reaction depending on multiple factors. What works for one patient may fail miserably for another, and there are no firm "right" and "wrong" answers. What's right for the individual is what works.

Some aches and pains, including most joint and muscle discomforts, are amenable to garden-variety analgesics such as the NSAIDs that are among the mainstays of treatment in the rheumatic diseases; they're discussed in detail in Chapter 4 and should be taken only with your physician's concurrence.

More stubborn muscle and joint pain may be amenable to physical therapy (PT), and your rheumatologist—or an orthopedic consultant to whom your regular doctor may have referred you—may prescribe such treatment. Physical therapists are highly trained professionals, often with superior knowledge of anatomy and bodily mechanics, who focus on both pain relief and prevention of future discomfort. Their techniques may include massage, the application of ultrasound and other modalities, heat and/or cold, and a variety of exercises and other routines designed to relax, realign, and strengthen as needed.

When a series of PT sessions has ended, most therapists will gladly provide instructions for continuing at-home exercises that will keep the benefits coming. One of the electromechanical techniques used in professional PT, called *transcutaneous electrical nerve stimulation* or TENS, can also be continued; many patients have purchased TENS units for home use (they are available from medical-supply firms and from a number of online sources) and have found them quite helpful.

Headaches, too, may prove amenable to treatment with NSAIDs and other common analgesics—but, depending on the kind and intensity of the headache, they may not. So-called "tension" headaches may have multiple causes—muscular and/or neural, perhaps with an overlay of mental or emotional stress as well—and so may require more than one remedy.

Migraine headaches are so prevalent among lupus patients—perhaps 10 to 15 percent suffer from them—that some clinicians consider them a significant part of the lupus signs-and-symptoms spectrum, although they're unmentioned among the diagnostic criteria. Migraine actually constitutes more of a syndrome than a mere headache, typically involving a constellation of symptoms, and requires special treatment. The family of focused drugs called triptans—sumatriptan (Imitrex), eletriptan (Relpax), zolmitriptan (Zomig), and others—are often helpful when NSAIDs prove inadequate, as are some agents in other classes of drugs not specifically designed to treat migraine; among the latter is topiramate (Topamax), an antiseizure medication.

In cases of especially stubborn headache of whatever apparent kind, a rheumatologist or primary-care physician will often feel that referral to a neurologist is wise in order to confirm and clarify the diagnosis before proceeding to further treatment. Headaches can be deceptive and may signal other problems, from tumors to (more commonly) dental infections to food or drug reactions; they may also be atypical, with associated symptoms predominating over the headache itself (visual distortions or gastrointestinal upsets, for example, in the case of migraine). Sorting out these diagnostic dilemmas may require special tests and other procedures and lies within the province of the neurologist.

When pain of any kind proves especially resistant and it's been established that no acute infection, malignancy, or the like is involved, the patient may be referred to a special multidisciplinary facility dealing solely with pain management. Typically, such a team practice uses the combined approaches of the physician, who can diagnose and who can prescribe medication if needed; the physical therapist; and the psychologist, who can help to sort out emotional components and is versed in such approaches as relaxation programs.

Medications prescribed to counter pain aren't limited to those that may come to most patients' minds as pain relievers; certain other classes of drugs have been found valuable for this purpose as well. All are powerful drugs. None should be combined with other drugs except on a physician's explicit direction. None should be combined with alcohol.

The potent synthetic narcotics are employed, if necessary, and they are useful, but they are not a first resort. Such drugs are known as opioids, that is, opiate-like; they include, among others, hydrocodone, propoxyphene, tramadol, meperidine, and oxycodone. Among the host of products containing such drugs, alone or in combination with acetaminophen or aspirin, are Darvon, Demerol, Endocet, OxyContin, Percocet, Roxicodone, Tylox, Ultram, and Vicodin. They are potentially habit-forming—addicting—and they are prescribed, and should be taken, with great caution.

Also employed to deal with pain are some of the medications traditionally viewed as aimed at emotional difficulties such as stress, anxiety, and depression. Perhaps that's not really surprising when we consider the universal recognition, in recent years, of the physical roles of the nervous system and neurohormones in conditions once considered purely "psychological."

Sedatives and relaxants, sometimes called "tranquilizers," have long been used for this purpose, since they encourage rest and repose and tend to unclench tense muscles and connective tissues. Some, with minimal drowsiness effect, are intended for daytime use, others for taking at bedtime. They include a wide range of products, some differing from others only in very slight chemical variations or duration of action; drugs in this general class include triazolam (Halcion), zolpidem (Ambien), clonazepam (Klonopin), lorazepam (Ativan), oxazepam (Serax), buspirone (BuSpar), and others. As with many classes of drugs we've mentioned, some of the seemingly pointless multiplicity is truly helpful: A patient may respond well to one medication when another, very similar one has proved useless for that individual.

Some of the antidepressants have proved to be particularly effective analgesic agents, a hitherto unanticipated facility seemingly separate from their primary purpose; they may act directly as pain modulators, effecting an actual change in the individual's pain threshold. The dosage required is often lower than that for treating depression. Major modern antidepressants include a class called (from details of their chemical structure) tricyclics, as well as the newer and now more widely prescribed products that control the circulation of various neurohormones. Among the latter are bupropion (Wellbutrin, also marketed as the stop-smoking drug Zyban), trazodone (Desyrel), venlafaxine (Effexor), and the selective serotonin reuptake inhibitors (SSRIs), which include fluoxetine (Prozac), paroxetine (Paxil), citalopram (Celexa), and sertraline (Zoloft).

While both the newer and older groups of antidepressants may be helpful in treating pain, two of the older group, the tricyclics amitriptyline (Elavil) and nortriptyline (Aventyl, Pamelor), have proved particularly useful in coping with a condition called *neuropathy* and its accompanying pain, *neuralgia*—suffering or disease (*-path-*) affecting a nerve (*neur-*) and causing pain (*-algia*). Peripheral neuropathy, affecting nerve endings in the outer parts of the body (often in the feet or legs), is not uncommon in lupus and is frequent in diabetes.

A particular kind of nerve pain, *postherpetic neuralgia* (PHN)—the neuralgia that follows herpes zoster—can prove particularly agonizing and intractable; it may afflict many of those who have suffered through a bout of shingles, which strikes a substantial number of lupus patients. Amitriptyline or nortriptyline seems to help in about three in five cases.

Yet another kind of drug designed for a different purpose has also been found effective against neuropathic pain generally and PHN in particular: anticonvulsant medications, drugs to control seizures in people with epilepsy. One such medication, gabapentin (Neurontin), is now widely prescribed for PHN and appears to work well. (It has also occasionally been used for migraine.) Some patients report an initial reaction of unaccustomed sleepiness, but that seems to dissipate after a day or two. A second, similar drug, pregabalin, was reported in 2003 to have performed comparably well in clinical trials but at this writing has not received FDA approval for marketing.

HOW ABOUT IMMUNIZATIONS?

Lupus patients may be particularly susceptible to infection—especially if they are taking corticosteroids or immunosuppressants—and should protect themselves as much as possible. Sensible precautions include taking care of one's general health and, if possible, staying out of sneezing, coughing crowds. What about immunizations, routine and other?

For reasons that are obscure, the question has been somewhat controversial in some circles, and some patients report that their physicians have actually advised against immunizations. Such advice is misguided. There may be individual exceptions under certain circumstances; if you are pregnant, for example, or in the midst of a lupus flare, or taking certain medications, or undergoing dialysis, your physician may advise that particular immunizations are contraindicated. In general, though, lupus patients should receive the full complement of available immunizations, including influenza vaccine annually, a diphtheria-tetanus shot every ten years, and the vaccine against pneumococcal pneumonia if you're in the vulnerable group. Past concerns that these vaccines might trigger flares have not been borne out.

There have been some reports of a lower level of response to some vaccines in lupus patients, and your physician may want to do blood tests to be sure the level of protection is adequate; the pneumonia vaccine—usually given at five- or six-year intervals—may also have to be given more often, because the level of protection may fall unusually quickly.

The recently introduced nasal vaccine FluMist has at this writing been approved only for those between the ages of five and fifty; there are not enough data to confirm safety in younger children, and efficacy has not been established for older persons. It is *not* recommended for those with lupus or other chronic diseases, whatever their age; lupus patients should have the injection. Immunization is needed annually because the flu viruses mutate frequently, and the vaccine is reformulated each year to incorporate newly identified strains.

If for some reason you did not have the standard childhood immunizations or the diseases against which they guard—they include, in addition to diphtheria and tetanus, pertussis (whooping cough), measles, mumps, rubella, *Haemophilus influenzae* type b (it has nothing to do with flu but is a bacterium that causes meningitis, pneumonia, and other infections), chickenpox (varicella), polio, and hepatitis B— discuss with your physician the advisability of having them now. Some are more important than others. Pertussis, for instance, is a less severe illness with increased age, while rubella poses a particularly serious peril if it's contracted in pregnancy.

As to *non*-routine immunizations—that is, vaccinations for travel: For most diseases endemic to specific regions, vaccines are not generally considered necessary unless the traveler will be straying into remote or rural areas, which are probably best avoided. The wisest course would be not to plan trips to areas in which particular infectious diseases are either endemic or epidemic.

Current information on specific destinations, including disease risks and recommended protective measures, is available from the Centers for Disease Control and Prevention; see the section on resources at the back of the book.

NOTES

1. Not sure whether your weight is in the hazardous range? A value called the *Body Mass Index* will tell you. The simplest formula for finding it (there are several, all leading to the same figure): square your height in inches—that is, multiply that number by itself; divide that answer into your weight in pounds; finally, multiply by 703. The result is your BMI. If it's under 25, you're fine; if it's over 25 but under 30, that's a bit worrisome; 30 or higher takes you into the danger zone of definite obesity; and a BMI of more than 40 signals what medicine calls *morbid* obesity, a significant threat to your health.

CHAPTER

9

Tests, Trials, Trust:
Doctor–Patient Relations

Medicine is classed as a science, but it is far from an exact one. In some areas, there is little or no disagreement among its practitioners: All physicians would agree that smoking cigarettes is harmful to your health, that a bacterial infection is best treated with an antibiotic (they may not necessarily agree on *which* antibiotic), that it is wise to have physical checkups at intervals (they may not agree on *what* intervals).

Yet in many ways, medicine is more art than science. Physicians' experience, coupled with their philosophies and attitudes, may well affect how they choose to assess facts and apply scientific knowledge. Here are some observations on such matters and how they might affect the treatment of lupus—and more specifically, the lupus patient. That treatment depends very much on having a doctor on whom you can rely for both crisis management and, at least as important, continuing support.

FINDING A PHYSICIAN

Your physician is the person to whom you entrust your health. That means you should have full confidence in the physician's professional abilities *and* feel comfortable with his or her attitudes and approaches to you and to your illness. This applies in any patient–doctor relationship; it applies especially to lupus—a chronic, unpredictable disorder demanding a high degree of patient–physician teamwork.

If you have unexplained symptoms and you think you may have lupus, or your general internist or family physician suspects that you may have lupus, you should be referred to (or you should seek) a board-certified rheumatologist. A rheumatologist is a physician who has chosen to specialize in internal medicine and to subspecialize further in rheumatology, the branch of medicine dealing with lupus, rheumatoid arthritis, and related autoimmune and arthritic disorders.

Any licensed physician may develop an interest in particular parts of the body, classes of patients, or kinds of ailments and may then describe himself or herself as, for example, an orthopedist, pediatrician, or allergist. Such a physician may even possess above-average skills. "Board-certified" means that the physician not only has an interest in a specialized area but has also passed examinations attesting to his or her expertise. A board-certified physician, also referred to as a diplomate of the particular certifying board (in this case the American Board of Internal Medicine), will display—or can produce, upon request—a document to that effect. A board-certified rheumatologist will have received certification first in internal medicine and subsequently in rheumatology.

It's best if the physician deals with nothing *but* rheumatology; while practice may not always make perfect, it does lead to greater depth of knowledge and acquaintance with the spectrum of illness within that area.

How do you locate a qualified person if you haven't been referred by your primary-care physician? Two very good ways: (1) Contact the nearest major medical school or teaching hospital (hospital affiliated with a medical school); direct your inquiry to the department of medicine (in medical schools, that means internal medicine) and ask for several recommendations. (2) If there is a chapter of the Lupus Foundation or the Arthritis Foundation in your area, put the question to the people there; both should be familiar with the leading specialists in your area.

There are also some reliable resources on the Internet, both for locating specialists and for looking into physicians' credentials and affiliations. See the resources section at the back of the book. (Always use more than one source; Web sites, in particular, have been known to contain careless clerical errors, including misstatements of medical specialty areas.)

Aside from board certification, what should you look for in this physician with whom you are likely to have a long-term relationship? First of all, pay attention to what the *physician* wants to know about *you*. You are a unique individual. A good physician will not view you as Lupus Case (or Possible Lupus Case) Number 337 but as a human being experiencing health problems. The physician should want to know everything about you that might have a bearing on those problems, everything that might define them and lead to solutions.

You should, of course, receive a thorough physical examination. You should be asked for samples of blood and urine for analysis (other diagnostic tests, as well as X rays, may also be needed—and if you question the reasons for them, explanations should be forthcoming). And you should be questioned about:

- the symptoms and complaints that brought you to this physician, with attention to timing (when did they start? do they come and go? are they connected with particular times, places, or activities?);
- any other physical problems or changes you've recently experienced;
- whether you smoke;
- whether you drink, and how much and how often;
- recent weight gain or loss;
- any medications or supplements you take regularly or frequently, both prescription and nonprescription;
- your general lifestyle, including the work you do;

- your recent travel, especially outside the country;
- past major illnesses, injuries, and surgical procedures;
- any allergies or other chronic conditions;
- if you are a woman, your menstrual and reproductive history.

In some circumstances, the physician may also ask about medical histories of close relatives.

Then, you'll want to ask some questions of your own, especially relating to availability. Is someone on call when your own physician is on vacation, or attending a conference, or teaching medical-school classes, or coping with another patient's emergency? Who is that person? (Sometimes a group or associate practice, with patients' records readily available to each physician, is a good idea.) If you should need to be hospitalized for any reason, where would that be? (Depending on the community, physicians may admit patients to one, two, or more hospitals.)

The physician may volunteer something of his or her approach to treatment; if not, feel free to ask.

And you may want to consider other questions of a practical nature—convenience of transportation, for example, if you're choosing among physicians located at varying distances from your home. Does the doctor have a "telephone hour" when patients can call with routine, non-urgent questions?

Your own instinctive reactions will—and should—play a part, too. Are you more at ease with a female physician or with a male physician? Do you feel better with an older (presumably more experienced) doctor or with a younger (presumably more up-to-date) one? Neither of these presumptions, needless to say, is necessarily true, but they may affect your own comfort level.

Physicians, like other people, have personalities. Some are terse, others verbose. Some are brusque and matter-of-fact; others go out of their way to encourage and reassure. Some explain in detail; others talk in generalities. Patients, like other people, have preferences. Some like a take-charge, just-leave-it-to-me doctor; others would rather be privy to all the nitty-gritty details. Some grudge time spent in the doctor's office; others see those visits as valuable opportunities to explore concerns. Does this physician's style and personality mesh with yours? You need to decide for yourself whether you think you'll be compatible.

Should you be forced to choose between a physician of unquestioned experience and competence who scores low in congeniality, and a charming sort with questionable professional credentials, you'll be wise to opt for the former.

If you've been referred to a rheumatologist by your regular doctor, the rheumatologist may either undertake your treatment or report back with a confirmation of the diagnosis and recommendations for therapy; it depends on what seems best for you. Typically, especially if you don't have other major medical problems, your lupus will be managed by the subspecialist, who'll keep your regular physician informed.

ACTION, INACTION, AND LAB TESTS

There is a cardinal principle of the practice of medicine that is learned by every future physician in medical school, faithfully observed by most, but unfortunately occasionally forgotten by a few: *Primum non nocere*. This Latin phrase means, "First of all, do no harm." In lupus, in which severely disruptive drugs must sometimes be used to control or dispel severely destructive or debilitating disease processes, this prime directive often translates to, "Treat the patient, not the lab tests—and don't *overtreat*."

Laboratory tests do play an initially important part in establishing the existence of lupus, basically confirming a diagnosis the experienced rheumatologist has made on the basis of examining and talking with the patient. They may also be vital in ruling out *other* conditions—such as malignancies, endocrine malfunctions, acute infections, allergic reactions, physical injuries—requiring very different treatment. Further, initial lab tests establish "baseline" values for later comparison. And later, in the course of continuing care, they can be extremely useful in monitoring the effectiveness of a particular therapy.

Beyond those roles, lab tests are not necessarily terrific predictors of a patient's needs or prognosis. And they may not be good guides to optimal treatment in the absence of significant signs and symptoms.

The aim is to keep the patient as healthy as possible—which means, essentially, two things: controlling and relieving symptoms that interfere with the patient's enjoyment and quality of life; and preventing and coping with critically threatening complications, such as kidney disease. Lab-test results are not always indicative of the patient's status in either area of concern.

Indeed, there is often apparent contradiction between lab tests and how the patient is actually feeling and functioning. In many cases, patients with test values traditionally viewed as alarming—high erythrocyte sedimentation rate (ESR), low levels of serum complement, and high levels of anti-dsDNA antibodies—may remain perfectly well and free of complications with little or no treatment. Because lupus *does* present the threat of serious complications, both patient and physician must of course remain alert for worrisome signs or symptoms—but that needn't, and shouldn't, mean taking unnecessary drugs.

As we pointed out in an earlier chapter, very few lupus patients ever need to be hospitalized. Nor do a great many lupus patients need to be on the massive drug regimens on which they are, too often, placed. Some physicians seem to be unaware that a person who has lupus *need not necessarily be taking any medication.* Therapy should be keyed to symptoms—and even then, need not involve drugs.

Fatigue, for example, is often a prominent symptom. If it becomes totally debilitating, and nothing else works, medication may be needed. Frequently, however, another "prescription"—a combination of diet modification, rest, and a certain amount of specific exercise—will be wonderfully effective. Lupus is a condition in which disease activity, what lupus patients and their physicians call a "flare," is provoked by unknown factors including substances the patient may encounter in the environment. In such a condition, it makes little sense to introduce other potentially trouble-making substances unless they're clearly needed.

Nevertheless, medications *are* frequently needed to deal with discomfort or with disease that threatens vital functions. When medications are prescribed, your physician should indicate clearly how and when they are to be taken, for how long they should be taken, and any precautions you should observe, including interactions with foods and with other drugs. If there's anything you don't understand, ask.

THE ONGOING RELATIONSHIP

My regular doctor—well, actually, my gynecologist, who was the one I really saw sort of more or less regularly, at that point—referred me to a rheumatologist. I had these really odd mouth sores and a lot of fatigue, plus I was feeling kind of achy in a few joints, and she said she thought I ought to see a specialist, because I could have a connective-tissue disease.

He did tests, and he told me a test for being predisposed to blood clots was negative. Well, okay, I didn't have blood clots. And beyond that, he was very uncommunicative; I had to practically drag information out of him. And this was after I'd waited hours to see him. But I kept going back. I don't know why; there was always that long wait, and then he'd rush you out of the office. I saw him for about a year, trying different anti-inflammatories he prescribed, and finally I decided to change doctors, since not only did I not like him, but I wasn't feeling any better either.

I found another rheumatologist, and I had my records transferred to the new one. And my first visit was a real eye-opener. He came into the examining room, with a fat folder with my name on it under his arm, and the first thing he said was, "Ah, you have lupus." I said, "What? I thought I had rheumatoid arthritis." He said, "No, see, right here in your record: You have lupus." That first doctor hadn't even told me the truth about my diagnosis. Or else he was shuffling patients through so fast he wasn't sure who had what!

~

One of the things I really appreciate about my rheumatologist is that she realizes that a patient might benefit from other things besides strictly medical treatment, and she's up on the good people to refer to. She sent me to a great physical therapist, and I had some emotional problems around all this and she picked exactly the right shrink for me, too. She seems to understand her patients, not just their lupus.

Your continuing relationship with your doctor can be crucial to your health in a number of ways. Erosion of the relationship can cause you to question your physician's advice, rightly or wrongly—and to flout that advice, wisely or unwisely. It can cause you to deceive your doctor, intentionally or inadvertently. It can play havoc with communication between you and your doctor. If nothing else, it can upset you emotionally, and that is not something a lupus patient, or any patient, needs.

Your goal and your physician's goal are the same: to maintain an optimum state of health for you. The achievement of that goal requires, at the very least, mutual respect and honesty.

Respect, on the physician's part, means recognition of your independent status not only as a patient but also as an individual. Such recognition is evidenced by concern for your identity as a human being, including your occupational, parental, and other roles. It is evidenced by concern for your time: Although emergencies do occur, and some schedule disruptions are beyond the physician's control, patients should not routinely be kept waiting to see the doctor for inordinate lengths of time, in either the reception room or the examining room, whether as a result of careless disregard or of zealous overscheduling.

A respectful attitude also accords you dignified treatment: Your conversation in the doctor's office does not take place only with you unclothed on an examining table; there is subsequent discussion across a desk. And unless the physician is markedly your senior, you are not addressed by your first name unless and until permission is asked. (First-name usage should always be mutual.)

Respect is a responsibility of the patient, as well—again, in both a professional and personal sense.

Your physician wants what you want, your health and well-being, and is applying his or her knowledge and expertise to that end. Grant that effort the respect it deserves by following your doctor's carefully thought-out advice and instructions. (Failure to follow a physician's advice "cheats" only the patient.) Offer feedback, even if not specifically requested, as to how you're feeling (better? worse? the same?), your reactions to medication, whether new symptoms have appeared; only *you* can provide that information.

Respect your physician's working schedule by keeping appointments on time and advising the doctor's office promptly if something prevents you from doing so. Prepare for your visits with your doctor: Just as you expect your rheumatologist to review your chart (that's the medical term for your file) before your appointment, you should review *your* contribution to your meeting. Make notes on what you'll report about your symptoms, your responses to therapy, and so on—and any questions that have occurred to you. Recognize that your physician has another life—family, friends, recreational pursuits—as well and cannot be available to patients at all times; when you must consult with a substitute your doctor has selected, give the stand-in the same respect you would your own physician.

Honesty between patient and physician is absolutely vital and is really part of their mutual respect. That includes the physician's spelling out the patient's diagnosis frankly—or as frankly, the lack of one, if that's the case. Doctors—no matter how skilled, experienced, and intuitive—don't always know if an apparent flare signals something serious or is simply a transient episode of discomfort. Sometimes what's needed is not new or intensified treatment but heightened alertness on the part of both doctor and patient, to see whether the symptoms persist or abate; medicating in haste can sometimes do more harm than good. Help your physician to help you by using your own observational skills. Remember, always, that therapy in lupus is always very individualized; sometimes a period of careful trial and error, or simply watchful waiting, is needed, and *you* are an important part of that process.

Beyond that basic expectation of honesty on your doctor's part, how much information is provided may depend, to a degree, on your own wishes. Some patients are fascinated by medical minutiae; others prefer to be told only what they need to know and not to be burdened by complex scientific details. In either case, you deserve to be dealt with frankly and openly. Your questions should be answered to your satisfaction. If you express confusion or confess ignorance, you should receive clear explanations, not evasions or disdain.

By the same token, you must be honest with your doctor. That means answering questions—about your symptoms and feelings, about your habits and lifestyle, about your compliance with your doctor's advice and recommendations—fully and forthrightly. In fact, it's in your own self-interest to do so, since in great part, your input provides the primary "database" for your doctor's plan of therapy, especially in lupus. And don't ignore the little things—a brief bout of dizziness, unusual tiredness, a persistent headache—that might be insignificant but could, on the other hand, be valuable clues to your physician that something needs attention now—before it causes major problems later.

If you think you'd like to try—or you're just curious about—other kinds of therapy, *talk to your doctor about it.* Don't just quietly start "supplementing" your prescribed drugs with herbs from the health-food store, exotic bodily manipulations at the hands of a self-styled wonder-worker, or a mail-order "breakthrough" you've seen lauded on television or the Internet. Some "alternative" therapies may indeed be not only safe but potentially very helpful; others may be right for some folks but not for you; still others may be at best of dubious value and even downright dangerous. Discuss such possibilities with your physician first. Many doctors, to the surprise of many patients, are quite open to thinking outside the professional medical box. But your physician will also be aware of the need for careful consideration of any potential negative effects and can in some cases point out significant perils.

Even with the best efforts on the part of both patient and physician, some doctor–patient partnerships just don't work out. Never feel that you must remain with a particular physician. If you're not happy with the first rheumatologist you see (or you eventually become unhappy), seek another—or get another referral from your primary-care physician. Don't worry about hurting the deserted doctor's feelings; he or she will get over it.

Two important reminders:

(1) Don't forget that there are other specialists everyone must see regularly: an ophthalmologist for eye examinations; if you're a woman, your gynecologist for Pap tests (to detect incipient cervical cancer) and a clinic or other facility for mammography for early detection of breast cancer; your dentist for checkups on your oral health.

(2) Always make sure that every physician and dentist you see knows what the others have prescribed. Various medications may interact dangerously with others, rendering them either more or less potent; can have side effects that could be confused with symptoms of illness; and can distort the results of laboratory tests. It's vital that any doctor you see be aware of these possibilities. If you change physicians, take with you to your new doctor a full list of your medications—names, dosages, schedule—and ask specifically whether you should continue to take each medication. This conversation needs to take place because it's possible that your new physician may assume that you've abandoned prior prescriptions when you haven't—or that you are just starting treatment. *Assume nothing,* and don't let your doctor do so either. Your health is at stake.

CHAPTER

10

Day After Day: Coping

Your rheumatologist and other health professionals, with their professional advice and prescriptions, are indispensable to your coping with lupus, its recurring sieges and its occasional nasty surprises. But, while they may be on crisis call around the clock, they can't be with you always. The rest of your life—dealing with the challenges large and small on a day-to-day basis, doing what you can to make life a little less unpleasant, a little easier and, yes, healthier too—is up to you. In this chapter, we offer some thoughts about ways to meet and manage those challenges—about *living* with lupus.

SUNLIGHT AND OTHER LIGHT

I'd heard about it, but it had never happened to me before. I went to a picnic yesterday, and it wasn't even that sunny; we were partly in the shade—and today, I'm really sick. It's not just that I have a rash all over my face and arms. I have a headache, I'm sick to my stomach, I'm so tired and hurt so much all over that I can hardly move. I don't understand how sunlight could do all that.

✦

*Is it possible that the sun can do something to you in fifteen min-
utes? I swear, I wasn't out more than that the other day, and it
was only to the car, which was parked two doors away. I take
that walk every day, and I'm fine. But some days, all of a sudden, that butterfly rash is back—well, mostly butterfly; it's around
my mouth and the sides of my jaw, and on my neck, too.*

At least a third of people with lupus are photosensitive; sunlight, and some other light as well, can trigger not only skin reactions but even full-fledged flares of the disease. How ultraviolet light sets off this process is not well understood, but the fact that it can do so is well documented. By and large, lighter-skinned people are more apt to be photosensitive, but that isn't completely consistent.

At the 2003 scientific meeting of the American College of Rheumatology, researchers at the University of Pennsylvania announced that they believed they had found a particular variant gene responsible for causing photosensitivity. The gene appears to go into overdrive upon exposure to ultraviolet light, impelling skin cells into premature apoptosis, which is the name of the normal process by which each cell eventually goes into a winding-down phase leading to ultimate death (of that cell only); it's also called "programmed cell death."

That aberrant activity, in turn, often triggers the entire immune network into inappropriate response mode. The result: a burst of localized or even system-wide inflammation—perhaps just a rash, perhaps a full-blown lupus flare. The threshold—the exposure tolerance time—varies from one patient to another. Some patients find that it happens on every exposure, while others experience it only on occasion; the occasions are unpredictable.

Thus, lupus patients who are photosensitive and have systemic reactions, which could potentially lead to organ damage, are taking a serious risk if they don't take stringent precautions against exposure. That doesn't mean you need to go to the extreme of staying indoors with the shades drawn on sunny days. (Actually, clouds don't offer any substantial protection; they may block visible light to a great extent, but they aren't much of a bar to the damaging ultraviolet rays.)

Broad-brimmed hats and long sleeves are helpful (and you don't need costly "sun protection" costumes; any clothing that provides a mechanical barrier is fine). And the use of a sunscreen is a must, on *all* exposed skin. Sunscreens are rated by a *sun protection factor*, or SPF; the figure is a function of time lapse as related to minimal burning of the skin, and the higher the number, the longer the time skin can be exposed without burning.

Choose a sunscreen with the highest possible rating—and don't skimp. Sunscreens are formulated indoors under controlled-light situations; their makers cannot take into account every risk-increasing circumstance such as wind, heat, or altitude. Apply sunscreen generously and frequently, at least fifteen minutes prior to exposure, and always reapply it after swimming.

There are two types of ultraviolet light, varying in wavelength, known as UVA and UVB; the product should promise protection against both kinds. If you have a history of allergies, and many people with lupus do, you may want to look for a brand that doesn't contain paraaminobenzoic acid (PABA) or padimate, fairly common ingredients to which some people are sensitive.

Be aware, too, that reflected light can be just as damaging as direct light; light is especially strongly reflected from sand, water, and snow. Photosensitive lupus patients are probably smart to shun some places altogether, including beaches and boats, as well as golf courses, ski slopes, and other unshaded outdoor areas—summer *or* winter. And tanning salons, despite the safety claims they may make, are off limits as well.

> I'm sensitive to not only sunlight but also fluorescent lights. I can tolerate only about thirty minutes of sun, even with protection; I know that any more is going to make me sick. Fluorescents will do the same thing, but it takes longer, maybe an hour. So I can't work in an office that has only fluorescents. But I can go to other places, like restaurants; I just don't go to the ones that have that kind of lighting. Or if I have to do shopping in a store that does, I make sure I don't stay very long.

❧

I recently made a discovery: The light in the dentist's office acts just like sunlight with me, if I sit under it long enough. My last visit was a lot longer than usual, not especially painful or stressful, just longer because he was working on more than one area and several impressions had to be taken and there was a lot of just-sitting time. I was there about two hours, and the next day, sure enough: all-over pain.

Photosensitive patients ("sun-sensitivity" is a misnomer, since it's not just sunlight) should also avoid exposure to unshielded fluorescent bulbs, since they emit significant amounts of ultraviolet light, as do halogen lights. Other, less obvious sources, such as the intense working lights used by dentists, may also cause problems (ask the dentist to extinguish the light during waiting intervals to minimize your exposure). When in doubt, play it safe and apply sunscreen. In case you encounter dangerous or doubtful lighting unexpectedly, it's a good idea to carry sunscreen with you; some brands are handily available in portable sticks and wipes.

Any source of light is a potential source of trouble. Ultraviolet emissions may also involve ordinary office copiers, as evidenced by a case reported at an ACR meeting a few years ago, involving a lupus patient who had had repeated occupational exposure to copier flash lamps, with exacerbation of skin problems. Experimental testing reproduced the symptoms; a change in the occupational environment cured the problem and the patient's complications.

Finally, be aware that certain foods and drugs can increase photosensitivity. The foods that can do this are all plants containing chemicals called *psoralens*, which act, in the body, to potentiate the effects of the sun; prominent among them are lemons, limes, celery, parsnips, parsley, and figs. Some people who *don't* have lupus have even been known to suffer painful and unsightly skin eruptions when they've spilled lemonade on their skin on a bright, sunny day.

Among the drugs that can cause photosensitivity are some of the tetracyclines; piroxicam (Feldene), an NSAID; hydrochlorothiazide, a diuretic and antihypertension drug; as well as some sulfa drugs, anti-seizure medications, and antidepressants. Be sure to mention photosensitivity to any doctor who is prescribing a medication of any kind for you; there is almost always an alternative.

THE COSMETICS COUNTER

Speaking of skin: It's quite a miraculous organ. Partly, it's protective, shielding our insides from a frequently hostile environment. But substances can enter the body through the skin, as well. Indeed, pharmaceutical designers have in some instances deliberately used the skin as a portal for drug delivery. Among chemicals that have been administered to the inside of the body via patches placed on the outside are estrogens and other hormones, agents to allay motion sickness, relievers of chest pain in heart-disease patients, and most recently, nicotine to help smokers break the habit.

> *Until a few years ago, I had recurring bouts of joint pain, and nothing seemed to help. Then my rheumatologist said, "Why don't you try not coloring your hair?" Well, I did stop using the hair coloring. And I've had a lot less joint pain since then.*

In general, exposing our bodies to unnecessary chemicals is not a good idea, and that applies especially to lupus patients. Cosmetics are in that category. They contain many ingredients, not all of them tested; among those ingredients are a host of dyes, including tartrazine, a form of hydrazine. Nail lacquers contain sulfonamides. These are both agents implicated in causing lupus-like illness. A range of cosmetic preparations, including permanent hair colorings, can set off allergic reactions, to which people with lupus are often especially susceptible.

Not very many women—and women constitute the vast majority of people with lupus—can be persuaded to abandon cosmetics altogether. If you feel, as many women do, that appearing in public with no makeup at all is unthinkable, then at least use makeup very, very lightly and stay with one of the hypoallergenic brands from which substances most likely to act as allergens have been excluded. It may be especially helpful to avoid permanent hair colorings, which contain agents from the family of amines and have been definitely implicated in the activation of lupus. (Simple hair *lighteners* are safe.)

> I get the classic butterfly rash. With some lupies I know, it's just sort of a blush—but mine is really kind of an angry-looking red, and the skin is very dry and itchy. All the moisturizers I've tried just seem to make it worse, though.

> My rash was just on my face. Now, it's on my arms, too, and sometimes on my legs. My regular doctor sent me to a dermatologist, and she prescribed some stuff in a tube—some kind of steroid, I think. But it doesn't have any of those side effects you hear about.

Ordinary skin care can be a challenge with lupus, and the rashes and dryness that often plague lupus patients can complicate matters; if you also have Sjögren's syndrome, that, too, can contribute to overall skin dryness. Itching may signal an allergic reaction; if hands, arms, or legs are affected, that suggests contact allergy, that is, something that has touched the skin, something handled or perhaps (when the legs are affected) plants brushed against. But simple dryness can cause itching, too.

The basic rules here are (1) avoid anything, including cosmetics, that seems to provoke or aggravate the situation; and (2) engage in a little trial and error to see what might relieve the problem. And if itching is part of the problem, *don't scratch;* that can cause extremely unpleasant infections.

Most ordinary moisturizers—indeed, most cosmetics generally—contain perfumes, which can cause or exacerbate skin problems. Some sunscreens, as mentioned earlier, may also prove irritating to some people. Look for unscented, hypoallergenic products when you shop for any sort of cosmetics.

As to possible remedies: Plain calamine lotion may be helpful for itching. A number of 1 percent topical hydrocortisone creams are available without prescription (Bactine, Cortaid, Cortizone, Kericort); systemic side effects, common with the oral corticosteroids, are quite rare with the topical products. Warm baths with colloidal oatmeal or bath oil added at the end can be soothing—and pat skin dry; don't rub. Some people find glycerin soaps more soothing and less drying than the regular kind. If home measures and over-the-counter remedies aren't helpful, a consultation with a dermatologist may be in order.

Finally, a word about cosmetic *injectables*. One day, Americans, like those in many other cultures, may come to view facial folds and creases as signs of someone deserving of veneration. Until then, attempts to preserve the visage of youth will doubtless persist. Recent years have seen the growing popularity of a kind of nonsurgical cosmetic "surgery"—the injection of various materials into the skin to fill in or fend off wrinkling. There are two types: plump-up substances (collagen and the recently approved hyaluronic acid product Restylane) and botulinum toxin (Botox). The latter paralyzes expressive facial muscles. It is unwise to add stress to a body already under stress. It is especially unwise to actually insert unneeded foreign matter, risking unknowable hypersensitivity and hyperimmune reactions in the short or long term. Such procedures are best avoided.

SEXUAL ACTIVITY

The subject of sex is one that comes up in physicians' offices far less often than it should, resulting in a great lack of information that can lead to serious misunderstandings. Both certain medications and lupus itself can have distinct physical impact on sexual activities, impact of which patients—and their partners—should be aware.

Tranquilizers, which are sometimes prescribed to allay anxiety, can occasionally suppress orgasm. Knowledge of this fact can relieve "What did I do wrong?" worries. A man taking medication for hypertension may experience erectile dysfunction ("impotence")—though *not* orgasmic dysfunction (the two are controlled by different nerves); if a change to a drug without this unfortunate side effect is not possible, a couple may find gratification by other means than the traditional. Remember that stimulation, for both sexes, can also be provided through digital, oral, or other means. (How about the several drugs now available to counter erectile dysfunction? Maybe. The drugs are not for everyone and are contraindicated in patients with several types of circulatory and kidney dysfunctions, as well as those taking certain medications.)

Corticosteroids may cause a number of sexually relevant difficulties. One is decreased libido, or sexual desire (it's *not* personal rejection of the partner), and a little more effort may be required for arousal. Another is easy skin bruisability, suggesting the necessity of a gentler, kinder touch. A third may be osteonecrosis, usually involving a hip joint, which can be quite painful and can interfere with achieving a comfortable position for sexual intercourse (for a full discussion of this condition, see Chapter 5).

Raynaud's phenomenon afflicts some 20 to 40 percent of lupus patients, causing pain in the fingers (or toes)—generally in response to cold, but sometimes in reaction to sexual activity as well, because blood flow is diverted to the genital area. A warm room and a warm bath prior to sexual relations can be helpful—and don't lean on your hands during intercourse.

Almost all those with lupus have some joint pain at one time or another. Nonsteroidal anti-inflammatory drugs (NSAIDs) or other pain relievers prescribed or recommended by your doctor may help—and again, a warm bath preceding sex may be useful. Beyond that, some experimentation may be needed to find positioning that minimizes discomfort.

If there's knee pain, for example, avoid flexion, and don't put any burden of weight on the knees; if both knees are involved, avoid intertwining the legs, which will cause increased pain. If one hip, knee, or shoulder is affected, try lying on the side with that joint upward. All-over achiness might suggest achieving sexual gratification by oral or manual activity alone.

When pain, or potential pain, is a chronic presence, it brings with it two other inhibiting factors: There is fear of pain on the part of the patient and, less often expressed, there is fear of *causing* pain on the part of the patient's partner. Sometimes simple reassurance, in response to the latter concern, can be extremely helpful.

An open mind on the part of both patient and partner, with equally open discussion about both desires and discomforts, is the most valuable aid to satisfying sexual activity.

EXPECT THE UNEXPECTED

If there is one pervasive vexation for physicians and patients alike, it's probably the unpredictability of lupus. A few lupus patients can see the times of heightened disease activity coming; most, though, are taken by total surprise.

My flares are definitely travel-related. I'm fine when I'm home. But when I travel, I always forget and let myself get overtired. And I just know I'm letting myself in for a flare.

❧

I can tell when a flare is coming, because I get depressed. Well, actually, I don't really know if the flare causes the depression, or I get depressed about something and that brings on the flare. But they definitely go together.

❧

Absolutely the worst part of this disease is the unpredictability. You never know what's going to happen. There's no rhyme or reason to it. There's no way you can make plans. Sometimes I could swear a change of weather brings on a flare—but the next time, it's a totally different season and there isn't any change in the weather at all.

❧

I think I've got this thing under control. I'm feeling pretty good—well, considering. The meds are working. And then some little thing goes wrong in my life, and it's back—the fatigue, the pain from head to toe. Of course, I don't admit I've been hit by another flare. I just keep going. Or try to. Needless to say, that doesn't help.

❧

My biggest problem is that when a flare hits, I forget that it's temporary. I mean, I know it is, but I get so depressed when it happens that it feels like it's going to last forever. And I think feeling that way actually makes it worse somehow. So I get even more depressed. And I know I have to deal with it, which means getting some rest, so I call my sister to come and babysit. Then I feel guilty, and of course, that's depressing, too.

In the observation of physicians who treat lupus, flares often follow or accompany marked stress. Precipitating stresses can be physical, emotional, or a combination of the two. Many are completely unpredictable—an acute infection or injury, an adverse reaction to a medication, a sudden death in the family, the loss of a job, the breakup of a long-term relationship. But others can be anticipated. When patients demand too much of themselves, schedule too many work or social commitments, overload their schedules, foolishly (let's face it) engage in activities they know have caused trouble before, flares can follow.

There's no way to prepare for the flares that follow completely unexpected events. But lupus patients do need to be frank with themselves and acknowledge that this is a coming-and-going disease. There *will* be flares. If you avoid the triggers you've *recognized* as triggers—the overdoing, the overscheduling, the overcommitments, the known emotionally or physically stressful situations—then some, perhaps even most, of the eruptive episodes can be aborted.

One more thing: Don't smoke. Smoking isn't just bad for your heart and lungs. It's been shown to interfere with the therapeutic action of a number of medications, among them two of the lupus mainstays, the corticosteroids and the antimalarials. And research published in the *Journal of Rheumatology* in 2003 demonstrated a clear connection between cigarette smoking and lupus flares; the data, the investigators concluded, offer yet another reason that "individuals with SLE should avoid all exposure to tobacco products."

The reverse of the flare coin is, of course, remission. What does "remission" mean? Unfortunately, there's no medical (or other) specification of length of time or exact definition. For some patients, remission means a virtually disease-free state; for others, it's strictly a relative term meaning, "not so bad." Some remissions, for some patients, may last for years; for others, the respites last only for a few months or even mere weeks.

HOW TIRED CAN YOU GET?

The fatigue is just awful. You feel like a wet dishrag, completely helpless and powerless. You can't get rid of that feeling by just lying down for half an hour. This is a different kind of tired.

~&

People with lupus need a new word for fatigue, because it's not just fatigue as normal people understand it. It's as if you had been forced to stay up—on your feet—for three days straight.

The almost indescribable total tiredness goes by many names: "superfatigue," because it so overshadows all the common, everyday, garden-variety forms of fatigue; "wipe-out fatigue," because it seems to obliterate every ounce of strength, both physical and mental; "terminal fatigue," because what totally drained, utterly dysfunctional state could possibly lie beyond it?

There is no one cause of lupus fatigue, no single trigger that might be banished by a single drug. Several factors, varying with the individual (and not mutually exclusive), may be implicated in this extreme fatigue: a degree of anemia, not uncommon in lupus; increased secretion, often seen in lupus, of an adrenal hormone byproduct called etiocholanolone (it may also raise temperature); lack of "productive" sleep, due to joint discomfort or other factors, at night; the side effects of many medications; lower-than-normal blood levels of thyroid hormones or of essential minerals; and, not least, inflammation itself.

Whatever the reasons in any particular instance, this extreme exhaustion is a very real symptom of lupus and, like other facets of the disease, deserves treatment—a concept that can be difficult for many people, including people with lupus, to grasp. The treatment is *rest*, in whatever dosage is right for that individual. It is as important as any prescription medication.

> For some reason the fatigue hits me when I travel, usually the minute I get where I'm going, even if I've been doing absolutely nothing but sitting in a seat on a plane. I've learned that I simply must allow time for the equivalent of a good night's sleep on landing, whatever time of day it is, because only then will I be okay and be able to enjoy the rest of the trip. By that, I don't mean six or eight hours; I mean at least nine or ten. If you're a lupus patient, you have to learn to sleep when you need it.

❧

> My company lets me telecommute, which is great, because I can sort of arrange my day to fit my own needs, and they don't

care what hours I keep at home, as long as I deliver the ad copy on time. What happens to me when I'm having a flare is that I usually feel fine in the morning, so I take advantage of that. I get up really early and start my working day about 7:30, and I'm great until noontime. Then, after lunch, I go into my "coma." That's what I call it. It's a deep, deep sleep; I'm totally out, for two or three hours. It's an absolute necessity.

And every now and then, I decide I must have a day in bed. Maybe I'll decide the evening before, maybe that morning. When it's necessary, it's necessary. You have to let yourself accept that. But the acceptance isn't easy.

◆

Usually, I'm a very driven person. I just don't stop. Last year, I was going through a period where I had to have a lot of rest, and I had to cut my activity to what a normal person does. Mentally, it was very depressing. I'd come home and I couldn't even make dinner. But my family have been pretty wonderful. My husband's an extraordinary person, with his supportiveness and helpfulness around the house; he and my daughter just took over everything.

The "different kind of tired" often means that a different kind of rest is needed—different in both quantity and quality—along with other lifestyle adjustments. The notion that one's body has developed an entire set of new and unfamiliar rest-and-renewal requirements can be extremely disconcerting. But acceptance of that reality is essential. To deny it is to forgo a truly essential part of the treatment for lupus, one that only the patient can prescribe and administer.

My doctor warned me, "Don't live your life around your lupus." I understand what he meant; he didn't want me thinking like an invalid. Of course he's right, and I don't. But I had to be realistic. I owned a little antique shop, and I loved it. But I knew I just couldn't keep up with running a full-time business and take care of my health at the same time. I sold the shop.

That was the best decision I ever made. Now that I've gotten control of my life, I'm doing consulting work—appraisals, that kind of thing; I work maybe five hours a week, maybe ten or twenty, and I can take naps, or even sleep all day, whenever I want. I'm not letting lupus run my life, but I think I've adjusted to it.

BODY AND MIND

The biggest change in the way I live since I've known I have lupus is that I swim regularly. Before that, I'd been sort of on and off about exercise. I'd be good for a while; then I'd get lazy. But for the past year, I've been swimming as if my life depended on it—and in a way, I feel it does. I hate to say it, but everything they say about exercise is true: I feel more awake; I sleep well; I feel better physically; I'm more alert; I get fewer Raynaud's episodes and fewer flares.

Exercise—not marathon runs, not routines that challenge and stress and emphasize pushing the pain envelope, but moderate exercise that simply keeps inertia from setting in—is good. It's body-good and brain-good, as well; somehow, it triggers the release of endorphins.

The endorphins are neurohormones produced by the brain, and they bind to what we call opiate receptors in other areas of the brain. Those receptors are the same ones that would be targeted if you took an opiate or other powerful pain-killing drug, and the coined name of these substances reflects that; it's short for *endogenous* ("originating within") *morphine*. The endorphins—they're also generated during some other activities, including sex and some forms of meditation—act to diminish physical discomfort by raising the pain threshold, and they also promote a feeling of well-being.

And for people with lupus who are taking prednisone or another corticosteroid, exercise serves yet another crucial purpose: Exercise pro-
motes muscle strength that can help to counter the skeletal fragility
induced by steroid drugs.

What kind of exercise is best? It's a highly individual matter, depending on your capabilities and personal preferences, as well as what
will fit into your schedule and your life. If you like to exercise in the
privacy of your living room, along with one of the popular videotapes,
that's fine. Some people find group exercise works best for them, and
they attend aerobics classes.

Someone who's been very sedentary can begin by just walking
around the block, once each day; the following week, extend that
to twice around the block—or once around *two* blocks. That might
be coupled with the very simple starter plan suggested at the end of
Chapter 7. Bicycling is a good, all-around form of exercise. Swimming
is excellent, and for those whose joints are often achy, swimming in
a heated pool can be a wonderful form of simultaneous exercise
and pain relief. A physical therapist you've consulted for particular
joint or other problems can likely advise on the best kind of exercise
for you.

> *I used to take figure-skating classes at a local rink, and after my
> diagnosis, I kept going, because I could attend an early morning
> class, and that's when I feel best. Then the class time changed to
> mid-afternoon. That's my have-to-sleep time. I also used to go
> to a gym, but that got to be too much. I realized that I wanted
> and needed some exercise, though, so I got an exercise bike. I
> use aerobics tapes, too. My exercise time is when I feel best—
> the minute I get up in the morning, and I can do it at my own
> pace, without getting out and going anywhere.*

What else can help? As with exercise, whatever works for *you.*
Some lupus patients swear by transcendental meditation. Some say
that spending time in flotation chambers does wonders. Others have
ventured into disciplines such as yoga and tai chi—disciplines that

combine nonstress movement with an attitude/philosophy—and found benefits therein. There's no *medical* argument for or against any of these—although your own physician may feel that one or another will be more, or less, helpful for *you*.

Both the Arthritis Foundation and the Lupus Foundation have advocated tai chi (pronounced "tie chee") as a particularly good choice for those who suffer from joint discomfort. Developed some 250 years ago as a martial art, tai chi has evolved into a program of slow, gentle movements that only mimic such "fighting" disciplines as kung fu, with priority given to flexibility. The traditional movements may also be varied to accommodate particular physical needs and to avoid stress. Tai chi is taught in martial-arts schools as well as in many community centers and health clubs.

Exercise can strengthen your body and better your frame of mind, as well. There are also intangible, nonphysical resources to which some have turned with success.

Remember that emotional stresses, not just physical stresses, can cause flares. That phenomenon isn't confined to lupus but is characteristic of many chronic conditions. Multiple studies have documented an association between emotionally stressful events and sudden worsening of such disorders as hypertension, heart disease, peptic ulcer, asthma, and diabetes, among others.

The field of psychoimmunology is a young one, and largely unexplored, but we are beginning to understand that the psyche has a definite impact on the behavior of the immune system (as well as on levels of various hormones), although the mechanisms of this influence have not been fully mapped. Psychosomatic phenomena are very real; the word (which simply means "mind-body") does *not* denote something imaginary or "all in your head," nor does it imply that emotional responses *cause* the disease.

Sometimes, the person with lupus makes the connection; that's usually so when the source of the stress is clearly evident—when there has been a major event such as a move to a new home or a death in the family, for example. But when the patient is puzzled, short-term professional counseling may be helpful. Your physician can usually recommend someone appropriate, who may be a psychiatrist, a clinical psychologist, or a certified social worker.

Sharing your feelings and concerns with others who have similar feelings and concerns can also be enormously helpful, as many lupus patients have found. There are many mutual support groups—in person and online (now crossing international boundaries, thanks to the Internet)—who exchange information and experiences, relay news of research progress, and share hints and tips on helpful ways to deal with this disease's many facets. Local chapters may also hold informational workshops with physicians and other speakers who offer new insights on clinical questions and research. See the resource section at the end of this book for details.

CONSIDERING THE ALTERNATIVES

Probably most people suffering from chronic problems have wondered, at some point, about a variety of recourses loosely lumped under the phrase "alternative medicine" and meaning, broadly, just about any remedy your physician hasn't expressly prescribed or suggested. There are many such substances on the market.

Should you consider such possibilities? Many lupus patients have done so. In one survey of patients in the United States, the United Kingdom, and Canada, nearly half—49.8 percent—said that they'd tried such therapies; the 2000 report of the study appeared in the ACR journal *Arthritis & Rheumatism*. Certainly none of the alternatives should replace your own doctor's ministrations and advise. But how about turning to them as extras, as additions to your prescribed regimen? That depends.

Nonstandard therapeutic techniques and modalities. As previously mentioned, such disciplines as yoga and tai chi have been found to be physically helpful (and possibly psychically as well, to the extent that any good exercise program exerts that effect), whether or not you accept the underlying philosophy.

We've noted in another chapter that one traditional Far Eastern technique, acupuncture, may also be helpful for intractable pain. It *does* provide effective analgesia—though it has *not* been shown to cure or to modify underlying disease. Be sure, if you decide to try acupuncture, that it is administered by a trained, licensed practitioner; discuss the question with your physician, obtain an informed referral, and look into your state's licensing regulations. (There are, by the way, some individuals trained in both Eastern and Western medicine—who have both M.D. and acupuncture credentials.)

How about other techniques, such as hypnosis, or biofeedback, or other programs claimed to be possibly therapeutic? Since they *are* experimental, and no one knows whether they'll prove helpful or even whether they're safe, they're properly provided only under carefully controlled conditions. Such experiments should take place under the auspices of a hospital or other licensed medical facility or practice. The patient should not be asked to pay and, as a test subject, should be fully informed as to the nature of the experiment. If you hear of such experimental therapies, ask your physician about their validity. Current clinical trials of new therapies, including drugs in development, that are seeking subjects are also listed on the Internet (see the section on resources).

Vitamin and mineral supplements. Some such supplementary—or "complementary"—suggestions can be helpful. Many physicians feel that not only are the "recommended daily allowances" of most vitamins and minerals lower than the levels conducive to optimum health but that most people don't receive even those quantities of these essential nutrients from their diets. A daily multivitamin is probably helpful for most people, including people with lupus.

Additionally, some single-vitamin extras are often suggested for their patients by medical practitioners. Vitamin C is one of those, and many physicians—and periodontists, whose concern is gum disease—suggest supplementary vitamin C of at least 500 milligrams a day.

Whether extra quantities of other elements are called for depends on your particular situation. Extra helpings of certain B vitamins are sometimes suggested when there are heart or circulatory problems. If calcium is being taken for osteoporosis prevention, your doctor may want to check your vitamin D levels, since the vitamin is necessary for utilization of the mineral. But don't decide, on your own, to take mineral or single-vitamin extras without advice, since unneeded quantities of some of them could be harmful. That is especially true of the fat-soluble vitamins A, D, and E, which are stored by the body, but some others can trigger trouble as well.

Glucosamine, chondroitin, and MSM. A trio of substances often come to the attention of people with muscle and joint aches: glucosamine, chondroitin, and methylsulfonylmethane (MSM) are often sold in combination. These are substances that occur naturally in the body, although components of the manufactured products are in part produced synthetically, in part derived from various animal and vegetable sources. The products are claimed to help to slow the progression of, and ease the pain of, osteoarthritis and sometimes other conditions.

Are these compounds helpful? *Maybe.* Very few studies have been done, and the limited research reported so far suggests only that this kind of supplement *may* be helpful for osteoarthritis (arthritis that results from injury and/or "wear and tear") of the knee.

One of the reasons that research has been limited, however, is that, as with supplements generally, content is inconsistent (see further comment below). In one National Institutes of Health–sponsored study of glucosamine, chondroitin, and products combining them, no commercial source could be found to furnish a product consistent in content from one batch to the next; participating researchers had to compound it themselves. Similar difficulties have been reported by others.

In early 2004, a preliminary medical-journal report by researchers at Temple University resulted in news items suggesting that glucosamine might be able to enhance the pain-relief effects of the over-the-counter anti-inflammatory drug ibuprofen. It might, but what the consumer news items failed to mention was that the only experiments so far had been conducted in laboratory mice. Whether this happy result holds for humans remains to be seen; at this writing, the possibility is being pursued in clinical trials.

Other herbs and supplements.   Aside from that sort of product, which has special relevance for those with joint problems, there are a host of others purported to help you attain and retain optimum health—although their labels don't exactly claim that, because US law doesn't permit them to do so.

These products, which are found in many drugstores and in abundance on the shelves of "health food" emporiums, do not have the status of drugs but are classed as "dietary supplements." The law permits them to be marketed *without review or control* by the Food and Drug Administration. Fairly broad promotional claims are permitted, *provided* that a disclaimer is included stating that the product isn't intended to "diagnose, treat, cure, or prevent" any disease.

Although the makers of approved medications (both prescription and over-the-counter) have had their therapeutic claims, and their labels, reviewed and approved prior to marketing, that is not true of purveyors of supplements. They are required to list ingredients and to attest that such are safe, but it's entirely up to the government to turn up any mislabeling (after the fact), to pursue suspicions of dangerous content (also after the fact), and to uncover any related instances of serious adverse effects (with approved drugs, the manufacturers are required to keep tabs on, record, and report such incidents).

The bottom line is that the purchasers of these nostrums cannot possibly be sure of their content, let alone their effects and side effects. When serious harm to consumers has come to light from time to time and triggered investigation, some products have been found to include such substances—unmentioned on labels—as powerful hormones of various sorts; potent anti-inflammatories with major adverse effects; sulfas and similar drugs that might set off critical hypersensitivity reactions or interactions with prescription drug regimens. Alfalfa and other food substances are (especially in lupus and related conditions) common provokers of severe reactions—and may be contaminated. Between 1995 and 2002, seventeen outbreaks of *Salmonella* or *E. coli* infection associated with alfalfa sprout products were reported to the Centers for Disease Control and Prevention.

The fact that a supplement is labeled "natural," sounds familiar, or seems to have been around forever is no assurance of efficacy—or even safety. **St. John's wort**, for example, has not been proved particularly helpful for anything, and it has triggered severe photosensitivity in some people; it has also been shown to disrupt the beneficial action of other drugs, including medications used in the treatment of cancer and AIDS and in preventing transplant rejection. The benefits of **ginkgo**, for another example, are similarly unproved—and there have been a few reported cases of its causing bleeding. "Natural" estrogen sources—plants such as **black cohosh** (*Cimicifuga racemosa*) and **red clover** (*Trifolium pratense*)—may act as very weak estrogens (with insignificant benefit) but may also, paradoxically, have antiestrogen effects. **Echinacea**, promoted for use in minor infections, has provoked allergic reactions, including potentially lethal anaphylaxis, and some samples have been found to contain pesticides. It may also interfere with the action of immunosuppressants and is expressly contraindicated for people with autoimmune disease. **Kava** (*Piper methysticum*) carries a risk of life-threatening liver injury. Samples of the purported sleep aid melatonin have been found to contain unidentifiable contaminants. We could go on.

Online hype and hokum. With the advent of the Internet, there is need for a heightened index of consumer suspicion. The World Wide Web, which offers a vast and very welcome array of sound and valuable information (the resource section of this book points to many such sources), is also home to a similarly vast panoply of cyberscam and the twenty-first-century equivalent of snake oil.

Unlike stocks of packages on store shelves, Web sites are quickly and easily created and dismantled, and this sort of site is especially likely to demonstrate that ability. Instead of specific warnings about particularly outrageous instances that may have disappeared by the time you read this, here are some clues that should alert you to the probability that you've encountered a deceptive and possibly dangerous come-on; they're based, we regret to report, on observation of actual sites in existence at this writing.

- "Facts" that you know—from your reading and from legitimate sources—to be untrue, outdated, or inaccurate are cited.
- "Cure" is claimed for ills, including autoimmune diseases and malignancies, for which there is no known cure.
- The site links not to established foundations, universities, research groups, government agencies, and so on, but only to other fringe sources. (Links to legitimate sources, on the other hand, suggest that there is no fear of your learning the facts, or perhaps only that the seller is willing to gamble on your not following the links.)
- Sales seem to be the main aim and thrust of the site—sales of a product, an unusual therapy, and/or franchises or "training" for others wishing to join the sales network.
- A substance sold or recommended is claimed to cure or relieve a constellation of ills stemming from many different causes or unknown causes.
- Logic tells you that the substance being peddled is unlikely to be helpful in the treatment of the diseases cited; colostrum (the liquid preceding milk in nursing mammals) from cows, for example, is not useful in the treatment of flu, lupus, sinusitis, cancer, or AIDS; "magnetic mattresses" don't cure diseases.
- Therapeutic efficacy is claimed for assorted herbs and minerals, without credible evidence.
- Widespread deficiencies in diet, unsuspected by the general public and allegedly responsible for many ills, are claimed to exist (by someone offering to remedy them).
- It is asserted that a single glandular deficiency, such as growth hormone, is responsible for multiple difficulties—ranging, for

example, from muscle weakness to obesity, lupus, insomnia, poor skin texture, and low self-esteem.

- Testimonials from pleased customers play a major role.
- There are references to purported scientific reports, supporting the proprietor's claims, in professional journals—but few if any are publications you've ever heard of, and many seem to be published in other countries and languages.
- An unprecedented "breakthrough" or "miracle" is alleged to have occurred.
- Prescription drugs are offered for sale, but a prescription is not required—or prescriptions are offered, to be provided by physicians who have never met the patient.

CHAPTER

11

Lupus in Children and Teens

The subject of this chapter is *not* the newborn condition, called *neonatal lupus*, which may appear in a small percentage of babies whose mothers have lupus. That condition, typically associated with the antiphospholipid antibody syndrome, is usually transient, and you'll find details on it in Chapter 6.

"Regular" lupus in children and teens, like lupus with onset later in life, is a chronic condition. Symptoms, diagnosis, and treatment may differ, though not markedly, from those of the disease when it first appears in the twenties, thirties, or forties. There may also be significant emotional impact not only upon the growing child but upon other family members, siblings in particular. It's not at all easy for parents to cope with a child's or adolescent's chronic illness; lupus can prove especially difficult.

THE STATISTICAL PICTURE

Although not unheard of, lupus appearing before the age of five is extremely rare. After that age, the incidence gradually increases year by year through adolescence.

As in adults, more young females than males are afflicted by lupus, although the differences are far less dramatic. The ratio of girls to boys up to age ten is about three to one, according to most studies (some have estimated a lower ratio); that rises to six to one among adolescents.

There appears to be an even stronger familial association in child-onset lupus than with onset in adulthood. An estimated 27 percent of children with lupus—more than a quarter—have an affected first- or second-degree relative. Among children with lupus, a third of their parents and about 40 percent of their sisters have tested positive for antinuclear antibodies (ANA).

The concordance rate among identical twins—the occurrence of lupus in both twins—among children has been reported, in various studies, to range from 57 to 69 percent, a substantially higher proportion than that seen in adults.

The higher concordance is not unexpected, and it tends to support prevailing theory as to a genetic factor in lupus. Childhood twins—living in the same household, often sleeping in the same room, eating the same food, attending school together, and sharing other activities—are far more likely to be mutually exposed to the same viruses, the same air pollutants, and so on than adult twins. If lupus is triggered by a combination of genetic and environmental factors, that combination is much more likely to occur in childhood than later.

When both of a set of identical twins have lupus, though, it doesn't necessarily appear at the same time. In most cases, the second twin will develop the disease within about three and a half years, but reported intervals have ranged up to fourteen years.

SIGNS AND SYMPTOMS

Arthritis and rashes are among the most common first signals of lupus in adults, and that's true in children, as well. Most have a rash of some sort. Many complain of joint discomfort, and the joints may also be stiff and swollen.

About 50 percent of children—a somewhat higher proportion than among adults—have the classic butterfly rash across the nose and cheeks; some studies have reported a proportion as high as 75 percent. Other skin symptoms may include lesions of the discoid type (uncommon in children), crusty or scaly lesions (often mainly on the upper part of the body), and simple redness.

In youngsters, though, fever is also a major symptom—in fact, the most common. Overall, about 75 percent have an elevated temperature at the time of diagnosis; in some studies, the figures have been 90 to 100 percent.

Among other frequent symptoms are muscle aches, thinning hair or change in hair texture (it may become brittle), and enlarged lymph nodes ("swollen glands") in the neck, armpits, and/or groin. Still other symptoms may include poor appetite with consequent weight loss, headache, fatigue, Raynaud's phenomenon, and gastrointestinal problems. Children appear to be at greater risk than adults for kidney complications, and there is a higher incidence, among children with lupus, of blood abnormalities such as thrombocytopenia and hemolytic anemia.

DIAGNOSTIC DETERMINANTS

Children are generally subject to a host of infections and other disorders, and there is great theoretical potential for misdiagnosis. In one series of forty-some children with lupus described in the medical literature in the late 1960s, fully half had first been thought to have some other disease, often acute rheumatic fever (the diagnosis given for one in four) or rheumatoid arthritis. Other initial diagnoses that have been mistakenly applied in the past to youngsters later diagnosed with lupus include kidney infection, leukemia, epilepsy, mononucleosis, rubella, and infectious arthritis.

Now, lupus in children is much less likely to be confused with infections, cancers, and other conditions. Early and accurate diagnosis is now the norm.

No special tests or other standards just for children are employed in diagnosing youngsters. The American College of Rheumatology (ACR) diagnostic criteria—which are enumerated in Chapter 2—are applied to children, as well. In children as in adults, there are many cases of lupus that do not technically meet the official criteria, and other observations will also be taken into account. Reported results on key laboratory tests show no significant differences between children and adults.

LUPUS TREATMENT IN CHILDREN

It is best for a child with lupus to be treated by a pediatric rheumatologist, a subspecialist who is familiar not only with the disease but with children—and the ramifications of the disease in someone who is at the same time growing, developing, and changing both physiologically and psychologically.

Most of the same modalities used to treat lupus in adults are also used in therapy for youngsters—and, as with adults, the disease is unpredictable and treatment must be highly individualized to fit each young patient's situation.

Mild disease, manifested mostly by fever and minor aches and pains, can often be managed with a regular regimen of nonsteroidal anti-inflammatory drugs (NSAIDs), whether salicylates (aspirin and related drugs) or one of the many prescription medications. Hydroxychloroquine may be given for rashes and other symptoms. More serious or persistent symptoms may call for one of the corticosteroids or even an immunosuppressant. All of these standard lupus drugs are discussed in detail in Chapter 4.

Most of the complications seen in adult lupus, ranging from anemia to kidney dysfunction, may also occur in children—indeed, aseptic necrosis of bone has been reported to occur more often among youngsters taking corticosteroids than among adults—and the same recourses apply. In general—simply because children are, as a group, generally healthy as compared with adults—a child who does not encounter such complications as kidney involvement will generally do well, and children seem less likely than adult lupus patients to experience the overlay of other, non-lupus-related aches and pains. And if complications do occur, young people also tend to respond well to therapy.

Many children with lupus are sun-sensitive—the rate may be twice as high among children as compared with adults—and this becomes a special concern for parents, since children spend so much more time out of doors than adults. In individuals who are photosensitive, light can set off not only skin reactions, but systemic flares as well, so that—difficult as it may be—restrictions need to be imposed and preventive measures taken. See the guidelines and advice on this subject in Chapter 10, if they apply to your child.

One complication that can sometimes occur in children with lupus is premature atherosclerosis, an obstructive accumulation of fatty materials (lipids) in blood vessels. In 2003, a collaborative study began at Duke University in North Carolina and Stanford University in California to see whether the anticholesterol drugs called statins, used to lower lipid levels in adults, will prevent this buildup in children with lupus. The investigation, which is sponsored by the National Institute of Arthritis and Musculoskeletal and Skin Diseases (NIAMS), the division of the National Institutes of Health that deals with the rheumatological disorders, is called the APPLE trial, for "Atherosclerosis Prevention in Pediatric Lupus Erythematosus"; it involves several hundred children.

Parents should be aware that, as with adults, the prognosis for children with lupus has vastly improved over the past two to three decades. The survival figures are similar to those of adults, and some leading medical centers now report ten-year survival rates that approach 100 percent.

STANDARD PREVENTIVES

The major threat is often not lupus itself but infection, which is the most common cause of death in children with lupus. Children who have lupus are especially susceptible to infections if they are taking high doses of certain drugs. A sudden fever should alert a parent to a problem—which may be an infection, a flare of lupus, or something else; the bottom line is that the doctor should be called without delay.

It's important to realize that steroids, and immunosuppressants such as cyclophosphamide, lower the body's ability to resist infection. This means that it's vital for your child to receive all recommended childhood immunizations. Recommendations are issued by the Centers for Disease Control and Prevention (CDC) with the approval of the CDC's Advisory Committee on Immunization Practices, the American Academy of Pediatrics, and the American Academy of Family Physicians.

The present guidelines for routine childhood immunization include the following:

- Hepatitis B vaccine consists of three injections. The first is usually given before the newborn goes home from the hospital; the second, at one to four months (at least four weeks after the first); and the third, at least eight weeks later, generally some time between six and eighteen months.
- DTP (sometimes called DPT) shots protect against diphtheria, tetanus, and pertussis (whooping cough). There are five injections, given at the ages of two, four, and six months, at about a year and a half, and again at four to six years. After that, there should be a Td shot (the designation for the adult formulation, which drops the pertussis component) every ten years—at age fifteen, at twenty-five, and so on.
- Inactivated polio vaccine (oral polio vaccine is no longer used in the United States) is administered in a series of four shots given at two and four months, between six and eighteen months, and again at four to six years.
- *Haemophilus influenzae* type b conjugate vaccine (HbCV), sometimes called "the Hib shot," protects against bacteria that can cause a number of serious illnesses, including bacterial meningi-

tis (despite the name, there is no connection with influenza, which is caused by a virus). The schedule of injections starts at two months and may vary thereafter depending upon the brand of vaccine used; a total of either three or four shots is administered, with the last one given at about twelve to fifteen months.

- MMR, the measles-mumps-rubella vaccine, is given in two injections; the first shot is given at fifteen months, the second at either four to five years or at eleven to twelve years. The time of the second shot is dictated by local regulations and/or disease patterns. In high-risk areas, the vaccine may be given at one year, or a measles shot alone may be given even earlier (the MMR is still given at fifteen months).
- Varicella (chickenpox) vaccine, reserved a decade ago for children at special risk, is now a routine part of the immunization schedule for all children. The one-time shot is given at twelve to fifteen months (assuming the child has not already had the disease).
- Pneumococcus vaccine, another recent addition to the basic schedule, is given at two, four, and six months and again at twelve to fifteen months. The vaccine protects against the predominant bacterial cause of pneumonia in the United States as well as a leading cause of middle-ear infection in children; pneumococcus can also cause meningitis.

Your physician may suggest departures from this schedule; the reasons may include lupus complications, other illness, or a regimen of high-dosage steroids. Of course that advice should be followed. More important than the specific times mentioned (which are geared to the usual infant and child checkup visits) are the total number of doses and the intervals between them; if one shot in a series is postponed, then the next one may also be postponed to avoid an unacceptably short time between shots.

If you've realized, after reading the above rundown, that your child has missed any required immunizations, talk to your doctor about setting up a catch-up schedule.

In addition, your children *and* you should receive influenza protection each fall; see more about this important precaution below.

SPECIAL PRECAUTIONS

A rare condition called Reye's (pronounced "ryes") syndrome can strike children and teens and has been found to occur disproportionately often following a bout of influenza or chickenpox during which the child took aspirin. The syndrome, named for the Australian pathologist Ralph D. K. Reye, who headed the team that first described it in 1963, has a devastating impact on the gastrointestinal system, the brain, and other organs and is potentially lethal. Since the mid-1980s, the US Food and Drug Administration (FDA) has required that aspirin and products containing it bear labels warning that they should not be given to children and teenagers with chickenpox or flu; as a result, the incidence of Reye's syndrome has plummeted, to the point that some have trumpeted its "disappearance." The threat could reappear, however, if vigilance is relaxed.

If your child is already taking aspirin on a regular basis, making an effort to avoid flu and chickenpox (varicella) becomes especially important. As noted above, varicella vaccine is now a part of the standard childhood regimen; be sure your child receives it.

Chickenpox poses additional special risks in that it can under certain circumstances lead to truly critical complications, including pneumonia and encephalitis.

If an unprotected child who has lupus, or is taking aspirin-containing medication, or both is exposed to chickenpox—or to an adult with shingles, which is caused by the same virus—you should contact your doctor immediately; the child should receive immune globulin. If such a child actually becomes ill with what you suspect may be chickenpox—again, contact your doctor immediately about emergency medication.

As far as flu is concerned, everyone—including both adults and children, whether or not they have lupus—should receive vaccine.

The shots are needed annually and, since the several flu viruses mutate frequently, the vaccine is reformulated each year to incorporate all of the currently circulating strains. The flu season generally runs from November or December through March, and late October through early November is the ideal time for shots, since the protection lasts only a few months. It's a good idea for the entire family to be immunized. Your own physician will be aware of projections for a particular flu season and can advise on specific timing.

For those who hate needles and are within a certain age group, there is now an alternative. In 2003, the FDA approved a nasal-spray form of the vaccine (FluMist). It's quite a bit more expensive than the injectable form, but it may be helpful for youngsters as well as others who can't stand needles. It is recommended only for healthy persons between the ages of five and forty-nine—two doses six weeks apart for five- to eight-year-olds, one dose for those aged nine and up. Your doctor can tell you whether it's right for any particular family member.

As with varicella, there are antiviral drugs that can be used in case of exposure to, or infection with, flu under certain conditions. They are *not* substitutes for vaccine protection: They have not been shown to be effective against complications of flu, and they are not effective against all viral strains; nor has their efficacy been adequately demonstrated in very young children. They may nevertheless be helpful in an emergency. If you believe a family member at high risk may have caught the flu virus, see your doctor without delay.

PSYCHOLOGICAL AND EMOTIONAL CONCERNS

My daughter, age fifteen, was just recently diagnosed with lupus. She is now taking prednisone tablets. Her joints are hurting, she has anemia, and our doctor has warned us that her spleen will have to be removed. But the main problem is that her emotions and her temperament have really changed, and we are having a very difficult time handling this.

Adolescents are going through some very complicated transitions in many areas, including psychological and sexual maturation, social adaptation, and physical growth and development. It doesn't help to have a chronic illness, one that causes physical discomfort and is often unpredictable, superimposed on all that. In adolescents, prednisone may precipitate severe acne, obesity, temporarily delayed growth, and slowed sexual maturation, in addition to the distressing effects of the medication seen in adults. Extreme reactions are understandable.

In a situation such as this, it's wise to seek emotional support for both parent and teenager. Talk to your youngster's rheumatologist about your concerns; a referral for family counseling may be helpful. Or your youngster—especially if he or she is a teenager—may prefer to see an appropriate counselor privately; that wish should be honored. There are also support groups on the Internet geared specifically to teens, where kids can swap questions, answers, and concerns of all kinds.

With younger children, the main problem is often that they have no realization of the nature and seriousness of their illness. Especially when it is under control and they have no discomfort, they are heedless of the need for basic health-maintenance measures (eating properly to prevent nutritional deficiencies, dental hygiene, and so on) or for special precautions such as avoidance of overexposure to the sun—not to mention the necessity of following a medication regimen. That heedlessness is normal for kids, of course. When a child has lupus, parents need to take extra care to be sure the health rules are followed.

And do be prepared for personality changes. A young child who has a chronic illness may become difficult and demanding. A young child or teen may also react with rage, resentment, and rebellion, which may result, depending on the child's age and capacities, in behavior ranging from minor naughtiness to sexual promiscuity, illicit drug use, and other antisocial acting-out. Further complicating matters, corticosteroids can also trigger departures from your youngster's usual personality.

It might be wise to anticipate such reactions by seeking *preventive* psychological or psychiatric counseling, with a view to heading off incipient problems. If this is done before any problems arise, it need not appear to the child that such counseling is in any way a "punishment," or that the youngster has done anything "wrong." A visit or visits to a counselor can be presented simply as consultation with another doctor, who will bring another point of view to dealing with the illness of which the child is already aware; your pediatrician or family physician may be able to offer the best advice about such consultation. If a youngster can share his or her feelings about having this complex and confusing disease, perhaps those feelings can be steered into constructive channels before they explode.

If you have more than one child, you need to think, too, about the impact of the illness on the lupus patient's sibling(s) and on the relationship between them—as well as your relationship with your healthy child(ren).

Remember that, worried as you are about the child with lupus, and anxious as you are to take the necessary time to care for that child's special needs, the healthy child has needs, too. That child needs to know that your love and concern have not lessened because a sibling is ill. And remember that lupus is a chronic condition; this is usually not a temporary situation. Your child who has lupus needs to know that the illness does not and will not mean that the child deserves, or will receive, your exclusive attention.

Within the limits dictated by age, siblings should be given information about the disease, and its symptoms—which may be frightening or simply bewildering—should be explained. Young children sometimes view illness as a sort of stigma; they need to be assured that the sick child is not bad, is not being punished, and is not "abnormal." Do all you can to encourage them to continue to play and spend time together. Unless your doctor has advised you otherwise, there is no reason a child with lupus cannot (with sensible precautions such as sun protection) participate in sports and other normal childhood activities.

It's also helpful to discuss your youngster's lupus with teachers, coaches, and other adults in your child's life and to be sure they understand its ramifications.

CHAPTER

12

Of Known Cause:
The Other "Lupus"

Fred, a retired corporate attorney, and his wife, Ruth, had been enjoying their new life in Arizona for just about three years when it happened, in the early 1990s. They were transplanted New Yorkers, and Ruth, a freelance illustrator of children's books, continued her career, while Fred concentrated on his great passion, golf.

One day, as Fred strolled to the first tee, he suddenly fell to the ground, unconscious. The diagnosis was atrial fibrillation, a form of cardiac arrhythmia, or irregular heartbeat. Fred's internist referred him to a cardiologist, who prescribed procainamide, a drug that, taken daily, acts to stabilize the heartbeat. That seemed to solve the problem, and Fred returned to his golf game with confidence and enthusiasm.

A few months went by before it became apparent that something was amiss. The first clue was growing fatigue: "He complained of feeling tired all the time," Ruth recalled. Fred phoned his cardiologist, who seemed unconcerned. "I got no sympathy at all," he said. "He simply advised me to get more exercise—but I was much too tired to follow that advice."

Then, a week later, Fred fell. It wasn't renewed arrhythmia—his heartbeat remained strong and regular—and he didn't lose consciousness. "One leg just buckled under me, and I thought I'd just developed a trick knee. It happened again, and again. And then a fourth time—but I fell toward the other side; it was the *other* leg that buckled. And I thought, no, not *two* trick knees. It was about time for my annual checkup, so I made an appointment with my internist, and when I went for my exam, I told him about the problem."

Fred's general internist, unlike his cardiologist, was concerned. "He checked me thoroughly, and he found severe muscle weakness in both thighs. The muscles were just wasted. He said he suspected drug-induced lupus. He stopped the procainamide and put me on a different drug for the arrhythmia. He also prescribed a short course of pred-nisone. And he ordered blood tests, which confirmed the diagnosis."

Fred did fine on the new drug, and his doctor suggested physical ther-apy to help regain his muscle strength. Fred was able to put the experi-ence behind him, but Ruth looks back on it with more indignation. "Knowing what we know now, the cardiologist should have followed up. He should have responded right away to Fred's complaint of fatigue."

Ruth is right—not only because any physician should respond to a patient's report of a new symptom, but because the possibility of the complication Fred suffered should have come instantly to mind.

NOT QUITE THE SAME

The phenomenon has been familiar to experienced physicians for many years; it's known as *drug-induced lupus* or *lupus-like syndrome*—not the spontaneously occurring, chronic condition but an uncanny mimic—brought on by a specific agent, often an otherwise helpful, even lifesaving medication. It is not rare; there are probably well over 100,000 cases in the United States each year.

There are no established criteria for the condition. "Induced lupus" differs in significant ways from the naturally occurring disorder. One prominent difference is that simply because the drugs involved may be prescribed for anyone—young or old, of either sex—there is no typical patient demographic, as there might be said to be for lupus itself. Prob-ably, however, there are a disproportionate number of older males, because the more widely prescribed drugs that may trigger the syndrome are used to treat heart and circulatory ailments.

Often, there are only one or two symptoms. As in Fred's case, fatigue and weakness are frequently prominent; joint pain is often a significant complaint, as well. There may also be fever, headache, and/or pulmonary problems. Much less commonly, anemia or skin or kidney involvement may occur—but never central nervous system symptoms, which can occur in "regular" lupus.

Laboratory tests show both similarities and distinct differences. One of the lab tests in "lupus" induced by medications, the test for antinuclear antibodies (ANA), is nearly always positive—although it's *not* consistently positive in lupus itself. A test for antibodies to a widely distributed protein called histone is positive in a reported 90 to 100 percent of cases of the drug-caused illness, but in only 30 to 50 percent of actual lupus patients. Antibodies to double-stranded or "native" DNA (dsDNA) are found in 60 to 85 percent of lupus patients, but in fewer than 5 percent of those with the induced syndrome; in some studies, *no* patients have evidenced such antibodies. Nor do they have any of the "special" antibodies to extractable nuclear antigens frequently found in lupus—anti-Sm, anti-Ro, anti-La, and anti-RNP.

The main, and ultimately completely defining, difference between lupus and the drug-induced condition is that once the drug or other substance causing it is withdrawn, the illness abates (and will return if the stimulus is restored—a confirmation established in research but, of course, not normally done with actual patients). This doesn't necessarily happen overnight; symptoms, as well as any physical damage (Fred's muscle wasting, for example), may persist and require therapy. But the condition will not progress and is not chronic, assuming the precipitating cause is removed.

THE MEDICATIONS

Many drugs have been implicated in triggering lupus-like syndromes; indeed, more than seventy different drugs have been reported to be associated with such syndromes. (That is not necessarily proof of cause.) The one first prescribed for Fred's cardiac arrhythmia, procainamide (Procan, Pronestyl), leads the list; it triggers the syndrome in approximately one-third of those taking it. In addition to procainamide, hydralazine (Apresoline, and a number of brand-named combinations, prescribed to treat hypertension) and chlorpromazine (Thorazine, an antipsychotic and antinausea agent) are the best known of the "lupus" inducers, the ones with which physicians have had the most experience. Such a reaction was first recorded in the 1940s; the drug was a sulfonamide. Hydralazine was the second confirmed agent, in 1953, and procainamide the third, in 1962.

As older medications have been supplanted by newer agents, additional drugs have been implicated as potential triggers of the syndrome. Minocycline, a member of the tetracycline family of antibiotics, has emerged as a worrisome agent, as have the antituberculosis drugs isoniazid and rifamycin; some sulfa drugs, anticonvulsants, oral contraceptives, and cholesterol-lowering medications; and ironically, some of the newest, cutting-edge agents used to treat another autoimmune disorder, rheumatoid arthritis.

As with lupus itself, some people seem to be more susceptible to the drug-induced syndrome, and there has been speculation that, as with the "real" condition, there may well be a genetic connection.

That possibility underscores a particular observation: Some people break down, or metabolize, certain drugs in the body faster than other people. Involved in this process is an enzyme produced by the liver, called acetyltransferase. Individuals who metabolize the drugs in question quickly are known as rapid acetylators, and they have a relatively high level of acetyltransferase activity; those who take longer are called slow acetylators, and they have a lower level of enzyme activity. Whether one is a fast or slow acetylator is known to be genetically determined, and the US population is more or less evenly divided between the two types.

Drugs such as procainamide and hydralazine, which happen to require acetylation, can induce a lupus-like syndrome in both rapid and slow acetylators, but the time required is markedly different. One

study, for example, followed a number of patients taking procainamide for cardiac arrhythmia; after six months on the drug, all
the slow acetylators had developed antinuclear antibodies (ANA),
but only a third of the rapid acetylators had done so. The positive
ANA blood test is *not* necessarily predictive of the syndrome—although if it does develop, it seems to be more likely to develop in slow
acetylators, and it is likely to develop substantially earlier. (But the
time may still be months, or even a full year.)

Two points should be made about the acetylation phenomenon.

One is that although procainamide, hydralazine, and certain other
drugs linked to the induced syndrome require acetylation in the metabolization process, some others also known to trigger it do not. The
level of acetyltransferase activity is therefore not a consistent factor
in the occurrence of the drug-induced syndrome.

Second, the phenomenon may or may not have implications for lupus itself. It has *not* been demonstrated that there is a substantially
higher proportion of slow acetylators among people with lupus than
among the general population, although some investigators have suggested that the proportion is *somewhat* higher. Researchers working
with inbred strains of laboratory mice that spontaneously develop a
lupus-like illness have been exploring this question among others.

IMPLICATIONS FOR LUPUS PATIENTS

What do these observations mean for those who have "real" lupus?
Should—or *must*—all medications ever associated with drug-induced
lupus be avoided? Are they also potential aggravators of the disorder
itself?

No, not necessarily. Most physicians would carefully weigh such a
reported association against the potential benefit of the specific drug.
If a connection with drug-induced disease has been well documented
and appears to occur in a significant proportion of those who have
taken the medication, the prescribing physician is likely to choose
another therapeutic agent if more than one is known to be effective

for the condition being treated. In most cases (there are rare exceptions), there will be a choice. The guiding principle here is a well-known medical maxim: "Don't ask for trouble."

BREAST IMPLANTS

Finally, there is the disturbing question of silicone gel breast implants, still not fully resolved after more than a decade of controversy. In recent years, more than 200,000 American women have received implants annually (estimates for the year 2002 ranged from 225,000 to 236,000 women), 20 percent for clinically indicated reconstruction (following cancer surgery, injury, or some other disease or disorder that has caused disfigurement) and the remainder for cosmetic enhancement.

Although they had been in use since the 1960s, no definitive safety studies had ever been undertaken. A 1976 medical-device law giving the US Food and Drug Administration (FDA) authority over such implants "grandfathered" devices already in wide use, while reserving to the agency the right to demand answers should questions of safety or effectiveness later arise. It was only in 1988 that the FDA notified manufacturers of the silicone gel implants that evidence of their safety would be required.

Risks of the implants had long been known to include scar tissue and hardening; the possibility of the implant's obstructing cancer-detection imaging; and migration of gel outside an implant's envelope, with unknown impact on other parts of the body. By early 1991, a possible cancer link was reported—but to only one brand of implant, since withdrawn from the market, in which the silicone envelope was sheathed with a polyurethane foam.

Aside from the cancer question, the main concern has focused on reports of autoimmune disease, apparently resulting from the antigenic action of silicone gel, either leaked from intact implants or spilled when the envelopes ruptured. The syndromes were variously described as "like" scleroderma (skin thickening, a prominent characteristic of an autoimmune disorder, progressive systemic sclerosis, that may affect various parts of the body); "resembling" rheumatoid arthritis; or "lupus-like." In a few cases, conditions much like Sjögren's syndrome have been seen, albeit without the antibodies usually associated with Sjögren's (that is, anti-Ro and anti-La).

Several studies of women with silicone gel implants and symptoms suggesting connective-tissue disease were reported in the early 1990s. Symptoms included, among others, fatigue, joint pain, and Raynaud's phenomenon. Many patients elected to have the implants removed. (If the implants have leaked, and silicone has migrated to other parts of the body, removal of the implants may not necessarily end the symptoms.)

Not surprisingly, reassurances were issued by the makers of the products, typically acknowledging the research reports and even listing observed symptoms, but declaring that (in the words of a confusing statement by one major manufacturer) "It cannot be said with assurance whether silicone breast implants are associated with diseases of the immune system, or whether abnormalities in the immune system cause connective tissue disease."

In 1992, the Food and Drug Administration concluded that there were sufficient data to question the safety of the silicone implants, and the agency asked physicians to stop inserting them and manufacturers to stop supplying them, pending review by a special panel.

The review was conducted, and the panel of experts announced its finding that although the link with autoimmune disease was still inconclusive, the data failed to demonstrate the implants' safety. Rates of rupture and leakage, as well as the frequency of autoimmune disease to which silicone might be linked, could not be established.

The panel recommended that use of the silicone implants be restricted to patients admitted to clinical study projects, with the goal of answering those safety questions. All those wishing reconstruction following cancer surgery would be eligible, as would others with serious breast deformities, but the panel said that availability of the silicone implants for cosmetic purposes should be sharply curtailed. The FDA issued an order implementing the panel's recommendations, banning use of the silicone-gel implants for purely cosmetic reasons as well as establishing specific criteria in patient selection among those in other categories, including ages and medical histories (women who had been diagnosed with lupus or scleroderma, among others, were excluded). The physicians performing the implant surgery, said the agency, would be responsible for seeing that all criteria were met and for keeping comprehensive records. A number of long-term studies were launched.

We wish we could report that all of this had led to clear and definite answers. Unfortunately, it has led instead to a decade of conflicting conclusions.

In 1993, for example, University of California, Davis, researchers reported finding "unique" antibodies—specifically, to the connective-tissue component collagen—in women with the silicone implants. Then, in 1994, the *New England Journal of Medicine* published a study, by a Mayo Clinic team, of all of the women in one Minnesota county who had had breast implants over a twenty-seven-year period; they found no association between breast implants and connective-tissue diseases. A 1995 Harvard study backed the Mayo conclusions. Later that year, *FDA Consumer*, the agency's official magazine, continued to call "autoimmune-like" and "fibromyalgia-like" disorders "possible" risks of the implants.

Similarly contradictory reports continued to appear, and some theorized that perhaps the observed signs and symptoms shouldn't be thought of as scleroderma, or lupus, or any kind of known disorder at all but signified some new and unique disease. Still, the research continued (by 1995, the FDA had decreed that silicone gel implants could be used *only* in women willing to become study participants). Practicing physicians grew as bewildered as their patients: Should patients' complaints be taken seriously? Were they alarm signals or mere reflections of discomfiting news reports? Many lawsuits were contemplated and some were filed; several makers of implants left the industry to pursue less uncertain lines of work.

In 1996, another Harvard study, published in the *Journal of the American Medical Association*, basing its data on reports from women who were also health professionals, said that the data suggested "small increased risks" of connective-tissue disease among women with implants. Late 1997 brought a review of the situation by FDA officials, published in *The Lancet*. By then, diagnostic advances had improved the discovery of implant rupture, and even small leakages of gel were detectable with magnetic resonance imaging (MRI). But because those strides had not been paced by similar progress in pinpointing the consequences, the situation was still unresolved: "Women considering mammoplasty with silicone-gel breast implants cannot weigh the benefits and risks of this procedure until the magnitude of the risks is defined."

The studies, and the conflicting reports, continued. A March 2000 "meta-analysis" of published research over the years, by epidemiologists at the University of North Carolina, appeared in the *New England Journal of Medicine*. Its unsurprising conclusion: The analysts found "no evidence [with a single exception] . . . of a significantly increased risk of any specific connective-tissue disease, all definite connective-tissue diseases combined, or other autoimmune or rheumatic conditions." That not-very-helpful statement was followed by extensive comment on the assorted faults of the published studies, including their unstructured nature, dependence on memory, and possible bias, among other problems.

The following year, a panel undertook a similar review for *Arthritis & Rheumatism*, the journal of the American College of Rheumatology—with similar results. "No association was evident," said the group's report, "between breast implants and any of the individual established or atypical CTDs [connective-tissue diseases]."

Surely that would settle the matter? Perhaps—but perhaps not quite. Yet another review, by physicians at the Sheba Medical Center in Tel-Hashomer, Israel, appeared in early 2003 in the online *Cutting Edge Reports*. They, too, noted problems with many of the published studies, which were generally relatively small and not well controlled, and pointed out that several recent studies had simply not been included in the meta-analyses. They felt that a frequently high level of auto-antibodies in breast implant patients had in some cases been given short shrift. They suggested the need for larger studies, with particular attention to the possible roles of such factors as genetic pre-dispositions, as well as a barely explored possible association with the fibromyalgia syndrome, which has been recognized and defined only since the late 1980s.

Indeed, in an August 2003 statement, the Environmental Autoim-munity Group of the National Institute of Environmental Health Sciences noted that, "Although a causal relationship between sili-cone implants and systemic rheumatic disease remains unproven, a variety of local and systemic adverse events have been reported fol-lowing silicone implantation. . . . Further studies are needed to under-stand if silicone contributes directly or indirectly to these undesirable immune responses."

In October 2003, a special FDA advisory panel met to hear testi-mony, pro and con, on lifting the ban and permitting silicone breast implants to return to the market. Not unexpectedly, a prominent maker of the implants—which had continued to be available in Eu-rope and elsewhere—argued for permission (the company offered to accept a variety of monitoring, reporting, and educational condi-tions), as did the American Society of Plastic Surgeons; by and large, they and other advocates for lifting the ban urged a policy of in-formed choice with continued oversight.

Others, including some women's advocacy groups, felt the ban should continue until or unless safety of the silicone implants could be assured, or that the implants' availability should be unrestricted only for mastectomy patients and others with definite disfigurements, not for those desiring implants for purely cosmetic purposes; several prominent legislators shared that position. Patients appeared before the panel to bear witness on both sides of the issue.

After two full days of testimony, the FDA advisory group recom-mended that the agency permit the silicone gel implants to return to the market for cosmetic as well as surgical-reconstruction use, with a number of specific conditions, including the institution of a variety of consumer informational supports and additional training for physi-cians. Shortly thereafter, the physician who had chaired the advisory panel announced that he disagreed with the panel's conclusion and asked the FDA not to approve the implants' return to market. Early in 2004, the FDA declined to follow its panel's recommendation and advised the implant producers that it had revised its marketing application guidelines—saying, essentially, that it was not yet convinced of the implants' safety based on the information submitted up to that time. And that is where matters stand as we go to press.

If you are a lupus patient considering breast implants (of any type) for cosmetic purposes, you might think about the fact that it's probably unwise to stress the body with unnecessary surgery—or to have foreign objects (often potential triggers of unpredictable immune-system responses) implanted if they are not needed. Consider, too, that *any* breast implants may necessitate additional surgery for removal or replacement; may leave undesirable changes in appearance after removal, should that prove necessary; may adversely affect the ability to breast-feed; consistently make routine mammography more difficult to interpret, often necessitating additional or repeated imaging; and may affect the cost of health insurance.

IF YOU ALREADY HAVE BREAST IMPLANTS

Probably only in a minority of cases, among those thousands of women who have had silicone implants, have complications occurred. Ruptured or leaking implants may have to be removed. Although ruptures are minimally detectable by mammography (breast X ray), it should not be used for that purpose, since it exposes healthy breast tissue to unnecessary radiation and is, in any event, not the most accurate technique. Ultrasonography can be helpful. MRI scanning is the technique of choice for accurate confirmation of suspected rupture.

As previously noted, no one really knows how often leaks or ruptures occur. Estimates of rupture rates alone have ranged from less than 1 percent according to manufacturers to as high as 25 percent and more in some reports from physicians. There is no need or reason to remove silicone gel implants that have caused no problems and have not leaked or ruptured.

If you have breast implants, whether saline or silicon gel, you should take some special precautions:

- Have regular breast examinations by your physician.
- Be familiar with the appearance and feeling of your breasts, and see your physician immediately if you observe or experience any change.
- Promptly report any unusual symptoms to your physician, whether or not you believe they may be related to your implants.
- Have a mammography for the detection of breast cancer at the intervals recommended for women in your age group (if you have had breast-cancer surgery, consult your physician about the necessity for mammography).
- Realize that, as we've mentioned, implants can interfere with mammography by casting a "shadow" on the X-ray image, and any scarring can also distort the image. Implants also prevent the compression of the breast to the degree necessary to obtain a high-quality mammogram. This is a serious concern, since statistics show that survival rates are dramatically higher when breast cancer is detected at an early stage (that is, when the size is still very small).

Be *sure* that your mammography facility has personnel trained and experienced in imaging breasts containing implants; double-check when you make an appointment—and when you have a mammogram, be sure to tell both the technician and the radiologist that you have implants.

Accept any recommendation you may receive for repeat or enhanced imaging following standard mammography, such as ultrasound, MRI, or other computerized imaging techniques. Such additional investigations are offered for your protection; they do not necessarily signal trouble but are suggested when initial "regular" X-ray images are for any reason unclear or ambiguous.

13

On the Horizon:
Future Therapies?

The major medications used to treat severe and stubborn facets of lupus are discussed in Chapter 4. None is ideal; all bring adverse effects along with their benefits. There is a continuous effort to refine those approaches, to focus therapy more concisely so as to minimize harm, to find variant, less toxic versions of those drugs.

At the same time, other approaches are also being explored. Some are close to approval for clinical use; others are quite experimental; still others are only theoretical therapies, notions inspired by encouraging developments in the animal-study laboratories. Here are some that appear to hold promise.

HORMONES AND ANTIHORMONES

With the prominence of lupus in women and major incidence during the childbearing years, there has been sustained interest in the significance of hormones in general, and estrogens and other reproductive hormones in particular (see the speculation in Chapter 3). Not unexpectedly, researchers have wondered over the years: If hormones play some causative role, might they—or perhaps substances countering them—play a role in therapy, as well? Two such substances have recently attracted researchers' attention.

Bromocriptine. As mentioned in Chapter 3, some investigators have reported abnormal levels of the pituitary hormone prolactin in lupus patients of both sexes. The hormone plays a key part in encouraging milk production following childbirth; it's also called lactogenic hormone. (Prolactin is produced by both sexes but appears to have no significant role in males.) Unusually high levels in women at *other* times may be associated with some cases of persistent infertility due to absence of menstruation and ovulation.

A drug called bromocriptine (Parlodel), which acts to diminish the release of prolactin, has been used to treat that condition and others in which prolactin levels are inappropriate. Researchers have found that high prolactin levels in lupus appear to stimulate the production of autoreactive antibodies; thus, they suggest, bromocriptine may be useful in treatment. Thus far, results of limited human trials (following prior positive results in the mouse lupus "models") suggest that bromocriptine is about on a par with hydroxychloroquine for treatment of mild lupus symptoms and thus may indeed have therapeutic potential.

Prasterone. A synthetic hormone that has been in development for many years appears likely to receive FDA approval very soon as an adjunctive to corticosteroids in the treatment of lupus. Its name is prasterone (Prestara; in Europe, Anastar), and it is a synthetic version of an adrenal androgen (male hormone produced by the adrenal glands) called dehydroepiandrosterone, or DHEA.

Interestingly, DHEA is a precursor of testosterone *and* the female hormones estradiol and progesterone, and it is produced in both sexes—although men normally have higher levels than women; as noted in Chapter 3, DHEA levels are often below normal in lupus patients of both sexes. That observation led to the theory that perhaps administration of DHEA or some variant of it might be beneficial, and that idea led to the development of prasterone. As with most proposed lupus drugs, it underwent initial testing in the "lupus"-afflicted laboratory mice before clinical trials in human lupus patients commenced in 1993.

Prasterone (early on, known simply by the code designation "GL701," should you happen to encounter preliminary research reports, and for a while called by the trade name "Aslera") appears to be a welcome addition to the lupus pharmacopeia. In extensive studies over the past decade, it dealt well with multiple lupus signs and symptoms, decreasing the occurrence of flares and effecting general improvement confirmable by both patients and physicians, and by laboratory assessments as well. Prednisone dosages can often be significantly decreased, and by 2000, a secondary benefit had been noted in research reports: increased bone mineral density, with some reversal of steroid-associated osteoporosis. (A confirmatory trial specifically examining that effect was initiated in 2003, and final FDA approval, pending at this writing, is contingent on the results.)

Reported side effects are few and dose-related and appear not to be serious or irreversible; they may also vary from one patient to another and seem to be associated with individual "sensitivities" to the hormonal impact. They include a mild acne-like dermatitis (especially in premenopausal women), light hirsutism (facial hair growth), scalp hair loss, skin oiliness, and breast tenderness (especially in postmenopausal women); some patients have also reported heightened libido.

Important warning: Do *not* confuse this prescription medication with over-the-counter "dietary supplements," sold through various channels, purporting to contain DHEA. Typically marketed as "miracle drugs" or "superhormones," these products often come with an array of claims, suggesting that they will help to combat aging, promote weight loss, improve memory, stave off cancer, fight infection, and/or prevent heart disease.

Using such nostrums is a rather poor idea, for a number of reasons. Before a major treatment product can be marketed in the United States, it must undergo extensive testing for both safety and efficacy; the "supplements" are untested. Although there is stringent regulation of approved drugs (both over-the-counter and prescription), including labeling accuracy and product quality standards, "dietary supplements" are unregulated. There is no guarantee of either content or purity. The claimed main ingredient may not be present at all; if it is, there is no assurance of its strength or bioavailability. Other, possibly quite harmful substances may be included. And in the unlikely event that such a product were to be the equivalent of an approved drug, no hormone or similarly powerful medication should ever be used except when the need has been established, and the remedy prescribed, by a physician.

THE DMARDS

It's the immune system that goes awry in lupus, and so it makes a good deal of sense to look into possible ways to put it right, to try to temper the activity that turns it from trusted defense to self-attack. And, of course, the aim is to do so without weakening the system generally and imperiling the body's ability to resist the assaults of infectious agents. Drugs that do this—drugs designed to zero in on, and interrupt, the disease process itself (as opposed to dealing with symptoms such as inflammation)—are known as disease-modifying antirheumatic drugs, DMARDs (pronounced "DEE-mards") for short. A number of DMARDs are now used in the treatment of rheumatoid arthritis; although none has yet been approved for lupus, several are under active consideration.

Monoclonal antibodies.   There is a therapy that has been studied for a number of years in experimental animals—specifically, the mice, mentioned a number of times in this book, that have served as laboratory "models" of human lupus—but has only recently been viewed as viable in humans: the administration of monoclonal antibodies. Treating those mice with antibodies to gene products of the mouse major histocompatibility complex (the mouse counterpart of the HLA locus in humans; see Chapter 3) has been shown to suppress several forms of autoimmune disease, including the mouse equivalent of lupus. (The antibodies are known as *monoclonal* antibodies, because each is cloned from a single antibody-producing cell.) The challenge has been to dispatch the harmful, inflammation-promoting elements in the immune system without decimating the helpful, protective ones as well.

One monoclonal antibody now under study, LymphoStat-B, entered clinical trials in 2002; it is specifically aimed at a protein known as B-Lymphocyte Stimulator, "BLyS" for short, which is believed to play a key role in goading the immune system into inappropriate hyperactivity. A research team representing nine university medical centers across the country reported at the 2003 American College of Rheumatology meeting that in initial trials, there was significant reduction in BLyS and in specific troublemaking B cells, as well as diminished anti-dsDNA levels in some subjects; the treatment, which is believed to have potential in both lupus and rheumatoid arthritis, seemed to be well tolerated, with no more adverse events in treated patients than in untreated (placebo) subjects.

A second monoclonal antibody is primed to attack another protein, an antigen called CD20, found on B lymphocytes. Rituximab (Rituxan, known as Mabthera in Europe) is already used in the treatment of a kind of cancer, non-Hodgkin's lymphoma, in which such cells proliferate, and it is under consideration for rheumatoid arthritis, as well as for lupus and for the antiphospholipid antibody syndrome (APS), which is often coincident with lupus. In some trials, combining rituximab with a standard immunosuppressant such as methotrexate or cyclophosphamide has enhanced its effectiveness. In general, there appeared to be a great deal of variation in response to the agent, with some patients, and some aspects of the disease, more responsive than others; trials continue, with the aim of refining the best approach.

Selective immunomodulators. Taking a slightly different tack, other researchers have sought to create unique chemical agents that would single out specific, known troublemakers—the autoantibodies associated with the most bothersome aspects of lupus. One such has been under development and has, at this writing, progressed to late-stage clinical trials.

Known until recently simply by the code name "LJP 394," abetimus sodium (Riquent) is a novel formulation aimed at taking out anti-dsDNA antibodies—which, as noted in Chapter 2, are highly characteristic of lupus and indeed may be unique to lupus. These antibodies are strongly associated with flares of the disease and especially with bouts of nephritis. Reports to date suggest that administration of the drug results in lowering levels of anti-dsDNA antibodies and that those reductions are correlated with decreased risk of renal flares.

THALIDOMIDE

Readers who have long memories—or are well read in medical history—may be startled. Yes, this is the same drug introduced in the 1950s and abandoned with some haste in the early '60s. An effective sedative/tranquilizer, thalidomide had seemed ideal for that purpose; unlike some other such drugs, it apparently posed no danger of accidental (or deliberate) lethal overdose. But it proved to have an unforeseen and thoroughly devastating effect along with its beneficial action: It was teratogenic (from the Greek *teras*, "monster," and the *gen-* stem that refers to birth). Several thousand horribly deformed babies were born in Europe before distribution of the drug was halted (it had never been marketed in the United States).

As a direct result of that sobering experience, the United States has since then had laws firmly in place requiring thorough testing of new drugs to assure safety in pregnancy if they are intended for use by women who are—or may become—pregnant. Failing such assurance, drugs are not banned but must be clearly labeled for nonuse by such patients.

Although thalidomide was withdrawn in Europe and was not approved for sale in the United States in the '50s and '60s, researchers never completely lost interest in it. There has been renewed exploration of the drug's potential, with limited trials conducted under stringent Food and Drug Administration (FDA) regulations. Women of childbearing age who participate in thalidomide trials, for example, must not only test negative for pregnancy but must also either practice abstinence or use two effective birth control methods, and must have pregnancy tests at frequent intervals while serving as a trial subjects.

Both additional benefits and additional adverse effects have emerged from further testing of thalidomide, and because the drug is so complex, both its marketing and its testing are being tightly controlled by public health authorities.

Thus far, thalidomide (under the trade name Thalomid) has been FDA-approved (as of 1998) only for a single use: treatment of a debilitating and disfiguring complication of leprosy called erythema nodosum leprosum. (Worldwide, there are 6 million sufferers from leprosy; about 7,000 are in the US) It may be prescribed, for that condition, only by certain authorized physicians, under rigidly controlled circumstances.

Other potential uses are being very cautiously explored. It appears, based on thalidomide's various demonstrated talents, that it may be useful not only as a sedative/tranquilizer but also in treating a number of other conditions: some skin and mucous membrane manifestations of such autoimmune conditions as lupus, Sjögren's syndrome, and scleroderma; other inflammatory dermatoses; Crohn's disease; the aphthous ulcers (canker sores) that are common in AIDS patients, as well as the extreme weight loss ("wasting") seen in that syndrome; and a variety of cancers.

Small clinical trials in these conditions have continued, in most cases with promising therapeutic results; thalidomide seems to be helpful, for example, in treating severe and stubborn skin involvement in lupus that has resisted antimalarials and other therapy. Unfortunately, more side effects have also emerged, in addition to the drug's demonstrated teratogenesis. Some of those are effects, such as sedation and weight gain, that might be beneficial in some circumstances but very undesirable in others. Other, definitely troubling sequelae have included allergic reactions, amenorrhea, and peripheral neuropathy that can be irreversible. The last is particularly disturbing, in that it seems to be unpredictable and independent of dosage.

Thalidomide is, in short, a potent and puzzling drug with apparently enormous potential for both help and harm. Part of the problem is that no one yet understands precisely how it works, and that's the challenge now being addressed. Once that riddle has been solved, the hope is that analogues can be developed incorporating the various benefits that thalidomide seems to offer—*without* the dreadful drawbacks.

A PROTEIN FOR RENAL RESCUE

When kidneys fail, as they sometimes do in severe lupus (as well as in a number of other conditions), the only "cure" is a transplanted organ. While awaiting that solution, the only recourse is usually dialysis, a tedious, time-consuming, costly, and uncomfortable process at best. An alternative would be welcome—ideally, one that would reverse at least some of the renal damage.

The human body, when wounded, tends to heal itself, and one of the substances it uses to encourage that process is a protein scientists have designated bone morphogenetic ("form-generating") protein 7, or BMP7 for short. Indeed, a laboratory-produced version of the protein has been used in patients with broken bones to hurry the recovery process along.

As it happens, BMP7 is also normally found in significant amounts in the human kidney. When the kidneys are prey to massive inflammation, as in severe lupus, healthy tissue is replaced by scar tissue, a process known as renal fibrosis. Now, researchers have found that—at least in mouse "models" of such renal injury—BMP7 can turn that process around and get regeneration of healthy tissue underway. Might the treatment work for humans? The possibility is being explored.

TOTAL LYMPHOID IRRADIATION (TLI)

The experimental technique known as total lymphoid irradiation (TLI) was singled out as a promising tactic in the first edition of this book, in 1993. Since that time, little has changed; TLI still isn't routine treatment—but it's still promising. In TLI, radiation is carefully beamed to lymph nodes and other tissues where lymphocytes—the white blood cells that generate antibodies—congregate. TLI has been used for many years in treating Hodgkin's disease and other forms of lymphoma (malignancies involving lymphatic tissues), and it has been found to be effective in those conditions.

TLI appears to suppress the antibody production that relies on helper T cells—that subclass of lymphocytes of which there is a relative overabundance in lupus. The result: diminished levels of ANA and anti-DNA antibodies. One drawback of this approach seems to be the possibility of heightened susceptibility to infections.

TLI—which has also been used to treat rheumatoid arthritis and multiple sclerosis (as well as in attempts to stave off rejection of transplanted organs)—is still experimental, because long-term safety and efficacy have not yet been established. The increased susceptibility to infections has been a concern (such infections have included recurrent bouts of shingles); even more worrisome, an increased incidence of malignancies has also been reported.

Perhaps TLI will turn out to be right for particular patients but wrong for others. The hope is that researchers will be able define the ideal TLI patient and sort out prospective candidates, selecting only those who'll be sure to benefit and rejecting those less likely to be helped and more likely to suffer harm.

PLASMAPHERESIS

The technique called plasmapheresis was first proposed in the 1970s as a possible treatment for lupus. It's based on a principle similar to that of dialysis, in which blood is circulated outside the body and potentially toxic waste materials are filtered out; dialysis performs mechanically, outside the body, a process that is normally handled by the kidneys.

Plasma constitutes about 50 percent of the blood; it's the fluid in which the blood cells—red cells, white cells, and thrombocytes (platelets)—are suspended. *Pheresis* is the medical term (from the Greek *apheresis*, "removal") for any procedure in which blood is withdrawn, a specific part of its content removed, and the remainder returned to the body. In plasmapheresis, a quantity of plasma is removed and replaced by an inert colloid solution.

This procedure temporarily reduces the number of antibodies, antigen-antibody complexes, and other troublemakers in circulation. In clinical trials, it has generally been performed several times a week over a number of weeks, usually accompanied or followed by administration of an immunosuppressant, alone or combined with prednisone. The technique has also been used experimentally for rheumatoid arthritis and has been found to offer some relief from pain and disability, but the effect has been short-lived.

While some physicians continue to believe that plasmapheresis holds promise for the treatment of acute complications of lupus, the results of therapeutic trials have been mixed. At this writing, plasmapheresis has been proved effective in only one lupus-related condition, thrombocytopenic purpura—subcutaneous "bruising" that results from abnormally low platelet counts. Thus far, it doesn't appear to effect any reliable improvement in renal disease or other aspects of lupus; some researchers feel, however, that expanding knowledge of the immune system may suggest different, more effective approaches to using the technique.

STEM CELL TRANSPLANTATION

You've doubtless read something of this cutting-edge therapy, based on the theory that young, not-yet-matured cells of various types, warranted normal and healthy, might be delivered to the body and trusted to develop into mature cells that will behave in normal, healthy ways, replacing diseased or misbehaving cells of their type.

The source of such new cells might vary—and might even be the patient, if the cells are treated in some way before being returned to the patient's body. That has been the approach with lupus: Stem cells are extracted from the patient's own bloodstream and bone marrow, "cleansed," and returned to the patient, who has been deliberately immunosuppressed to destroy remaining abnormal cells.

The procedure, also under consideration for rheumatoid arthritis, is called autologous ("self-related") hematopoietic ("blood-making") stem cell transplantation. It is delicate and risky. It has been undertaken, so far, not in large clinical trials but only on an individual-case basis, with very strict selection and treatment criteria, in patients with persistent, severe, organ-threatening disease that has been stubbornly unresponsive to standard heavy-duty therapies.

Reports from the United States and Europe on the small number of patients who have been treated with this technique since its experimental use began in 1997 have been encouraging, with most patients experiencing long-term remissions of disease, some for several years. In 2004, the National Institutes of Health announced the launch of a five-year prospective study to further assess this form of therapy.

Glossary

Note: Words and phrases in SMALL CAPITALS *will be found in this glossary. Specific drugs and medications have been omitted from this listing but are included in the index.*

acetylation   a step in the metabolization of certain drugs; the rate at which this process takes place may determine whether a drug is likely to cause a lupus-like syndrome.

acetyltransferase   an enzyme involved in ACETYLATION.

ACL   the abbreviation for anti-CARDIOLIPIN antibody.

ACR   the abbreviation for American College of Rheumatology, the professional organization of those physicians specializing in RHEUMATOLOGY.

ACTH   adrenocorticotrophic hormone; a hormone, produced by the pituitary gland, that stimulates cortisol production by the adrenal glands.

AFP   the abbreviation for ALPHA-FETOPROTEIN.

alopecia   abnormal loss of hair from the scalp.

alpha-fetoprotein   a substance produced mainly by the fetal liver; assessment of levels in the maternal circulation may reveal information concerning fetal development.

amenorrhea   absence of menstruation.

ANA   the abbreviation for ANTINUCLEAR ANTIBODIES.

androgens   the predominant male hormones.

anemia   a deficit in red blood cells.

antibodies   substances produced by the immune system in response to infectious agents or other antigenic stimuli.

anticardiolipin   an anti-PHOSPHOLIPID antibody associated with a variety of circulatory problems and with difficulties and adverse outcomes in pregnancy.

antigen   a protein that provokes ANTIBODY production by the immune system.

antigen-antibody complexes   units of bound-together ANTIGEN and ANTIBODY, typically producing inflammation.

antimalarials   a class of drugs originally developed to treat malaria, which have been found helpful in the treatment of lupus.

233

antinuclear antibodies (ANA)   ANTIBODIES that act against material from cell nuclei (cores); tests for ANA are often positive in connective-tissue diseases.

antiphospholipid antibody syndrome (APS)   a condition, involving ANTI-BODIES directed against particular substances in cell membranes, characterized by clotting within blood vessels; the antibodies include ANTICARDIOLIPIN and LUPUS ANTICOAGULANT.

aromatase   an enzyme that plays a part in hormone activity.

arteriole   a tiny branch of an artery.

arthralgia   pain in and around a joint.

arthritis   inflammation of a joint.

arthropathy   disease of a joint.

arthroplasty   surgical correction of a condition involving a joint.

autoantibody   an ANTIBODY that acts against the body's own tissues.

autoimmune disorder (or disease)   a condition often characterized by the production of AUTOANTIBODIES.

avascular necrosis (AVN)   NECROSIS due to diminished blood supply.

B cells   a subclass of LYMPHOCYTES that produce ANTIBODIES.

baseline values   numbers, such as those obtained from initial blood or urine tests, used for comparison with later ones.

Behçet's syndrome   an AUTOIMMUNE VASCULITIS that may overlap, or be confused, with lupus.

biopsy   removal of a small sample of tissue for microscopic examination.

bisphosphonates   a class of drugs used in the treatment of OSTEOPOROSIS and other conditions involving bone.

bone mineral density (BMD)   a measure of bone strength versus porosity.

bromocriptine   a drug inhibiting the release of PROLACTIN, a pituitary hormone.

BUN   the abbreviation for blood urea nitrogen, the proportion of nitrogen in a blood sample deriving from its urea content; an elevated value may suggest kidney dysfunction.

calcitonin   a thyroid hormone essential to the bone REMODELING process.

calcitriol   the active form of vitamin D.

cancellous bone   TRABECULAR BONE.

cardiolipin   a PHOSPHOLIPID found in cells lining blood vessels.

CBC   the abbreviation for COMPLETE BLOOD COUNT.

cellular casts   fragments of bodily substances such as HEMOGLOBIN; their presence in urine may suggest kidney disease.

chloroquines   a class of antimalarial drugs also used in the treatment of lupus.

collagen   a protein substance that is a major component of connective tissue in the joints and elsewhere.

compact bone   CORTICAL BONE.

complement system   a component of the immune system, consisting of a series of proteins that perform various actions in support of ANTIBODY activity.

complete blood count   analysis of the number of cells—ERYTHROCYTES, LEUKOCYTES, and THROMBOCYTES—in a quantity of blood.

concordant   having a particular characteristic in common; persons are said to be "concordant for" the trait in question.

congenital   present at birth.

core decompression   a surgical procedure for the treatment of OSTEONECROSIS.

cortical bone   a type of bone found primarily in the long bones of the arms and legs and constituting approximately 80 percent of the skeleton.

corticosteroid   any of a number of medications resembling cortisol, a hormone produced by the cortex of the adrenal glands; their effect is to inhibit inflammatory processes.

creatinine   a waste product of muscle activity, normally excreted in the urine; the creatinine clearance rate is a measure of kidney function. It should not be confused with *creatine*, a substance, produced by the body, essential to muscle contraction.

densitometry   a procedure to determine the measurement of BONE MINERAL DENSITY, used in the detection of osteoporosis.

DHEA   the abbreviation for dehydroepiandrosterone, an adrenal ANDROGEN.

dialysis   see HEMODIALYSIS.

discoid lupus (discoid lupus erythematous; DLE)   lupus limited to the skin, characterized by thick, reddish, roughly disk-shaped lesions, with residual scarring; formerly considered a separate disease.

discordant   differing as to a particular characteristic; the opposite of CONCORDANT.

dizygotic   originating from two different fertilized egg cells; dizygotic twins are fraternal (nonidentical) twins.

DLE   DISCOID LUPUS.

DMARD   the acronym for "disease-modifying anti-rheumatic drug"; it is pronounced "DEE-mard."

DNA   deoxyribonucleic acid, a component of cell nuclei and the substance of the genes that transmit hereditary information.

dsDNA   the abbreviation for "double-stranded DNA," the form found within the nucleus (core) of all human cells.

echocardiography   visualization of the interior of the heart by the use of sound waves.

embolus   a migrating fragment of a blood clot.

ENA   the abbreviation for EXTRACTABLE NUCLEAR ANTIGEN.

end stage   in reference to RENAL disease, denoting that point at which kidney impairment has become potentially life-threatening.

endocarditis   see LIBMAN-SACKS ENDOCARDITIS.

endorphins   substances, produced by the brain, that bind to opiate receptors and raise the pain threshold; coined from "endogenous morphine."

erythema nodosum   a form of VASCULITIS characterized by painful reddish
nodules; it may be secondary to a number of infections and may also
occur in reaction to various drugs, as well as in systemic disease.

erythrocyte   red cell, a type of blood cell.

erythrocyte sedimentation rate (ESR)   the sinking velocity of red cells
within a quantity of drawn blood; it may be elevated in a number of
AUTOIMMUNE and other conditions but usually indicates the presence
of connective-tissue disease, inflammation, or malignancy.

estrogens   the predominant female hormones.

extractable nuclear antigen   any of a number of specific ANTIGENS, found
within the nuclei (cores) of cells, to which a significant proportion of
persons with lupus—and certain other disorders—have demonstrated
ANTIBODIES.

false-positive   in reference to testing, erroneously suggesting the presence
of a disease or other characteristic.

fibromyalgia   a rheumatic syndrome predominantly affecting muscles and
connective tissue, not infrequently seen accompanying lupus.

first-degree relative   a parent, child, or sibling.

flare   a period of increased disease activity.

glomeruli; glomerulonephritis   the tufts that make up the kidney's filtering
apparatus; inflammation involving these structures.

glucocorticoid   CORTICOSTEROID.

graft   a transplanted organ or other transplanted tissue.

heart block   a condition involving heartbeat irregularities due to misfiring
of certain electrical signals within the heart.

hematologic   relating to the blood.

hematuria   a condition in which the urine contains red blood cells.

hemodialysis   filtering of the blood through a mechanical device to remove waste materials.

hemoglobin   the oxygen-transporting pigment of the blood; it is found in
the ERYTHROCYTES.

hemolytic anemia   ANEMIA due to abnormally rapid destruction of red
blood cells.

herpesviruses   a "family" of viruses, some of which are suspected of playing
roles in various AUTOIMMUNE diseases.

herpes zoster   shingles.

histocompatibility   compatibility of tissues, as between an organ donor and
recipient.

HLA system   a region, found on the sixth human chromosome, controlling a number of immunologic responses. The letters stand for "human
leukocyte antigen."

Hughes syndrome   ANTIPHOSPHOLIPID ANTIBODY SYNDROME.

hyperlipidemia   abnormally high levels of LIPIDS in the blood.

immune complexes   ANTIGEN-ANTIBODY COMPLEXES.

immunoglobulins   substances, produced by B CELLS, containing ANTIGEN-specific ANTIBODIES.

immunologic   pertaining to the body's immune-defense system.

immunosuppressants   agents employed to suppress the immune system (for example, in organ transplantation and in AUTOIMMUNE diseases) and to treat malignancies.

ischemia   localized ANEMIA due to obstruction of blood supply to the affected area.

ITP   the abbreviation for immune THROMBOCYTOPENIA, a PLATELET deficit caused by AUTOIMMUNE activity.

keratoconjunctivitis sicca   that aspect of SJÖGREN'S SYNDROME specifically involving the tear glands and accompanied by inflammation of the cornea and mucous membranes of the eye.

LAC   the abbreviation for LUPUS ANTICOAGULANT.

latex fixation test   a test for RHEUMATOID FACTOR.

LE-cell test, LE prep   one of the tests that may be used in the course of lupus diagnosis.

lesion   any pathologic abnormality due to injury or disease; often, but not necessarily, used in reference to the skin.

leukocyte; leukopenia   white cell, a type of blood cell; a deficit in such cells.

Libman-Sacks endocarditis   a condition, characterized by wart-like growths on the heart valves, that may be seen in association with lupus.

lipids, lipoproteins   fatty substances, including cholesterol and others, that may interfere with circulation by accumulating in, and blocking, blood vessels.

lumbar puncture   withdrawal of a sample of cerebrospinal fluid, the fluid surrounding the brain and spinal cord, for analysis.

lupus anticoagulant   an ANTIPHOSPHOLIPID ANTIBODY associated with a tendency to clot formation and with pregnancy loss.

lupus vulgaris   an obsolete term for cutaneous tuberculosis involving the face; there is no connection with the disease now known as lupus.

lymphocyte   a type of white cell especially active in the immune system.

lymphokines   infection-fighting substances produced by T CELLS, a subclass of LYMPHOCYTES.

magnetic resonance imaging   a noninvasive diagnostic technique using radio-frequency pulses, permitting three-dimensional visualization of various body tissues.

mammography   X-ray of the breast.

MCTD   the abbreviation for MIXED CONNECTIVE TISSUE DISEASE.

menopause   the cessation of menstruation; the constellation of hormonal and other changes occurring at this time of life, often referred to as "menopause," is properly termed the *climacteric*.

MHC   an alternate designation for HLA. The letters stand for "major histocompatibility complex."

mixed connective tissue disease   a condition, often relatively mild, meeting the diagnostic criteria for two or more such diseases.

monoclonal antibody   an ANTIBODY, derived from a single cell, directed toward a specific ANTIGEN.

monozygotic   originating from the same fertilized egg cell; monozygotic twins are genetically identical.

MRI   the abbreviation for MAGNETIC RESONANCE IMAGING.

myositis   muscle inflammation.

necrosis   deterioration or erosion—for example, of bone.

negative   in reference to laboratory testing or other diagnostic procedures, unremarkable; displaying no departure from normal, such as the presence of microorganisms, etc.; not having a particular characteristic or condition for which testing or examination has been performed.

neonatal lupus   a distinct newborn syndrome characterized chiefly by a transient rash and transient blood-test abnormalities.

nephritis   kidney inflammation.

nephrosis, nephrotic syndrome   a kidney condition characterized by excessive excretion of protein.

neuralgia   pain involving a nerve or nerves.

NSAID   a commonly employed acronym for "nonsteroidal anti-inflammatory drug"; it is pronounced "EN-sade."

NZB/NZW mice   a laboratory-bred strain of New Zealand black and white mice, naturally susceptible to a lupus-like disease, widely employed in lupus-related research.

organic murmur   a heart sound signaling a structural aberration.

osteoblasts, osteoclasts   cells involved in the process of bone REMODELING.

osteonecrosis   NECROSIS of bone.

osteoporosis   a state of skeletal fragility, which may be due to hormone or mineral deficiency or may be induced by certain drugs.

partial thromboplastin time   a test for the presence of LUPUS ANTICOAGULANT.

pericarditis   inflammation of the pericardium, the outer membrane surrounding the heart.

peripheral joints   those of the hands, arms, feet, and legs.

phagocytosis   the process of ingestion—by certain white cells known as phagocytes—of bacteria, cellular debris, foreign material, etc.

phospholipids   substances, found universally in cell membranes, that may stimulate the production of ANTIBODIES.

photosensitive   abnormally reactive to light, especially ultraviolet light.

plasma   the fluid in which the blood cells are suspended.

plasmapheresis an experimental therapeutic procedure in which a quantity of PLASMA is removed from the circulation and replaced by an inert solution in order to reduce the quantity of circulating ANTIBODIES.

platelet THROMBOCYTE.

pleurisy, pleuritis inflammation of the pleura, the membrane lining the chest cavity.

polyarthritis simultaneous inflammation of a number of joints.

postherpetic neuralgia lingering NEURALGIA following an episode of shingles.

positive in reference to laboratory testing or other diagnostic procedures, indicating the presence of microorganisms, departure from normal values, confirmation of a particular condition or characteristic for which testing or examination has been performed, etc.

progesterone a hormone, produced by the ovaries and the placenta, essential to sustaining pregnancy.

prolactin a pituitary hormone that stimulates breast enlargement and milk production.

proteinuria abnormal levels of certain proteins in the urine.

psoralens chemical constituents of certain plants which, if ingested, can heighten photosensitivity.

PTT the abbreviation for PARTIAL THROMBOPLASTIN TIME, a test for blood clotting.

pulmonary relating to the lungs.

pulse therapy the administration of "bursts" of a drug by intravenous injection.

Raynaud's phenomenon (or disease or syndrome) a condition characterized by abnormal paling and numbing of the fingers or toes, in reaction to cold or other stimuli, due to vasospasm (also known as "red, white and blue disease").

remission a period of abatement of signs and symptoms of a disease.

remodeling the cyclic process of bone resorption and rebuilding.

renal relating to the kidneys.

rheumatoid factor an ANTIBODY found in rheumatoid arthritis as well as in some patients with other disorders.

rheumatology the branch of medicine focusing on lupus, rheumatoid arthritis, and other AUTOIMMUNE and arthritic disorders; it is a subspecialty of internal medicine.

"rhupus" a condition having characteristics of both rheumatoid arthritis and lupus.

RNP the abbreviation for ribonucleoprotein, an EXTRACTABLE NUCLEAR ANTIGEN; its presence suggests immunologic disease.

salicylates a family of anti-inflammatory drugs, including aspirin and others.

Schirmer test   an assessment of tear-gland function, used in the diagnosis of SJÖGREN'S SYNDROME.

"sed rate"   ERYTHROCYTE SEDIMENTATION RATE.

sensitivity   in reference to diagnostic screening tests, the relative proportion of cases of a disease or other condition likely to be recognized.

sicca syndrome, Sjögren's syndrome   a condition involving dysfunction of various moisture-producing glands, prominently those producing saliva and tears.

SLE   the abbreviation for SYSTEMIC LUPUS ERYTHEMATOSUS.

specificity   in reference to diagnostic screening tests, the ability to distinguish a disease or condition from others.

SPF   the abbreviation for sun protection factor, a rating of the efficacy of sunscreen preparations.

SSRI   the abbreviation for selective serotonin reuptake inhibitor, a category of antidepressant medications.

statins   drugs designed to lower the levels of LIPIDS in the circulation.

steroid   in the context of this book, short for CORTICOSTEROID.

subacute bacterial endocarditis   an infection of the heart valves.

systemic   affecting the body as a whole; not localized to one area, organ, or type of tissue.

systemic lupus erythematosus   the full medical name of the disease generally referred to simply as lupus.

T cells   a subclass of LYMPHOCYTES.

testosterone   the predominant male hormone.

thrombocyte   clotting cell, a type of blood cell.

thrombocytopenia   a deficit of THROMBOCYTES.

thrombosis   clot formation within a blood vessel.

total lymphoid irradiation (TLI)   the irradiation of lymph nodes and other tissues in order to suppress ANTIBODY production.

trabecular bone   bone with a lattice-like structure, characteristic of the spine.

tricyclic   a class of antidepressant medications.

undifferentiated connective tissue disease (UCTD)   a condition manifesting signs and symptoms of one or more such diseases but meeting the diagnostic criteria for none.

uremia   an excess of waste materials, normally eliminated by the kidneys, in the blood.

varicella   chickenpox.

varicella-zoster virus (VZV)   the HERPESVIRUS that causes chickenpox and shingles.

vasculitis   blood-vessel inflammation.

vasospasm   spasmodic occlusion of small blood vessels.

verrucous endocarditis   LIBMAN-SACKS ENDOCARDITIS.

xerostomia   dryness of the mouth.

Selected Look-Up and
Keep-Up Resources

Note: Omissions do not imply any opinions or judgments regarding sources not included. All information here was correct at the time of publication, but the reader should be aware that addresses, phone numbers, and Internet addresses may change. Relevant additional information may often be obtained through links from Web pages and by seeking referenced firms and institutions through general or specialized search engines such as Google (http://www.google.com) or Science Search (http://www.scirus.com).

ACUPUNCTURE

American Academy of Medical Acupuncture
4929 Wilshire Boulevard, Los Angeles, CA 90010; (323) 937-5514
http://www.medicalacupuncture.org/

US State Laws Regarding Acupuncture
http://acupuncture.com/StateLaws/laws-right.htm

ANTIPHOSPHOLIPID ANTIBODY SYNDROME (APS)

Arthritis Foundation, *Bulletin on the Rheumatic Diseases*
http://www.arthritis.org/research/Bulletin/Vol52No3/Introduction.asp

eMedicine
http://www.emedicine.com/med/topic2923.htm

Healthlink (Medical College of Wisconsin)
http://www.healthlink.mcw.edu/article/921732376.html

Hughes Syndrome Foundation
The Rayne Institute,
St. Thomas' Hospital,
London SE1 7EH;
(020) 7960-5561
http://www.hughes-syndrome.org/

University of Illinois
http://www-admin.med.uiuc.edu/hematology/PtAPS.htm

ARTHRITIS:
SEE RHEUMATIC DISEASES

AUTOIMMUNE DISEASES

American Autoimmune Related Diseases Association
22100 Gratiot Avenue,
East Detroit, MI 48021, and
750 17th Street NW,
Washington, DC 20006;
(586) 776-3900 and
(202) 466-8511; (888) 856-9433;
literature requests (800) 598-4668
http://www.aarda.org/

BONES

American Academy of Orthopaedic Surgeons
6300 North River Road,
Rosemont, IL 60018;
toll-free (800) 824-2663
http://www.aaos.org/

National Institute of Arthritis, Musculoskeletal, and Skin Diseases
http://www.niams.nih.gov/hi/topics/avascular_necrosis/index.htm

National Osteoporosis Foundation
1232 22nd Street NW,
Washington, DC 20037;
(202) 223-2226
http://www.nof.org/

Osteoporosis and Related Bone Diseases/ National Resource Center (NIH)
http://www.osteo.org/

CHRONIC DISEASES, DISABILITIES

Centers for Disease Control and Prevention
http://www.cdc.gov/nccdphp/ bb_arthritis/index.htm

Invisible Disabilities Advocate
http://www.myida.org/

National Center on Physical Activity and Disability
http://www.ncpad.org/

Women with Disabilities
http://www.4woman.gov/wwd

CLINICAL TRIALS

CenterWatch
http://www.centerwatch.com/main.htm

National Institutes of Health
http://www.clinicaltrials.gov/

Clinical trials are also listed in *Lupus Now*, magazine of the Lupus Foundation of America.

DRUG-INDUCED "LUPUS"

Arthritis Foundation, *Bulletin on the Rheumatic Diseases*
http://www.arthritis.org/ research/bulletin/vol51no4/ 51_4_drug-induced.asp

DRUGS, MEDICATIONS, SUPPLEMENTS

American Society of Health-System Pharmacists
http://www.safemedication.com/

Arthritis Foundation
http://www.arthritis.org/conditions/ DrugGuide/drugindex.asp

ConsumerLab (supplements)
http://www.consumerlab.com/

Food and Drug Administration
http://www.fda.gov/search.html

Medline (National Library of Medicine)
http://www.nlm.nih.gov/medlineplus/ druginformation.html

Memorial-Sloan Kettering (herbs, vitamins, supplements)
http://www.mskcc.org/mskcc/html/ 11570.cfm

National Center for Complementary and Alternative Medicine
http://nccam.nih.gov/health/alerts/

Over-the-Counter Medications
http://www.bemedwise.org/

Prescription Meds
http://www.drugs.com/
http://www.rxlist.com/

FIBROMYALGIA SYNDROME

Arthritis Foundation
http://www.arthritis.org/ conditions/diseasecenter/fibromyalgia/ fibromyalgia.asp

Fibromyalgia Support (Canada)
http://www.ncf.carleton.ca/ fibromyalgia/

National Institute of Arthritis and Musculoskeletal and Skin Diseases
http://www.niams.nih.gov/hi/topics/ fibromyalgia/fibrofs.htm

National Fibromyalgia Association
2200 North Glassell Street,
Orange, CA 92865;
(714) 921-0150
http://fmaware.org/

National Library of Medicine
http://www.nlm.nih.gov/medlineplus/ fibromyalgia.html

HEALTH/MEDICINE NEWS AND INFORMATION (GENERAL)

Agency for Healthcare Research and Quality
http://www.ahrq.gov/

Department of Health and Human Services
http://www.hhs.gov/

Digital Librarian (links)
http://www.digital-librarian.com/ health.html

Food and Drug Administration
http://www.fda.gov/opacom/ hpwhats.html

Google Health (daily)
http://news.google.com/news/en/ us/health.html

Health A to Z
http://www.healthatoz.com/

HealthDay News (daily)
http://www.healthday.com/

Intelihealth
http://www.intelihealth.com/

Merck Manuals (reference)
http://www.merck.com/pubs/

Morbidity and Mortality Weekly Report
http://www.cdc.gov/mmwr/

National Institutes of Health
http://www.nih.gov/

National Library of Medicine
http://www.nlm.nih.gov/

Quackwatch (frauds, scams, alerts)
http://www.quackwatch.org/

IMMUNIZATIONS

Centers for Disease Control and Prevention
http://www.cdc.gov/nip

LABORATORY TESTS (INFORMATION ONLY)

LabTests Online
http://www.labtestsonline.org/index.html

University of Washington
http://www.orthop.washington.edu/arthritis/living/labtests/01

LUPUS: ADVOCACY, RESEARCH, INFORMATION, FORUMS, AND MESSAGE BOARDS

Alliance for Lupus Research
28 West 44 Street, New York, NY 10036; (212) 218-2840 or toll-free (800) 867-1743
http://www.lupusresearch.org/

Arthritis Foundation
http://www.arthritis.org/conditions/diseasecenter/lupus.asp

But You Don't Look Sick
http://butyoudontlooksick.com/

Cleveland Clinic
http://www.clevelandclinic.org/arthritis/treat/facts/lupus.htm

The Doctor Will See You
http://www.thedoctorwillseeyounow.com/articles/other/sle_22/index.shtml

European Lupus Erythematosus Federation
http://www.elef.rheumanet.org/

Lupus Around the World
http://www.mtio.com/lupus

Lupus Canada
18 Crown Steel Drive, Markham, ON L3R 9X8; (905) 513-0004; toll-free (in Canada) (800) 661-1468
http://www.lupuscanada.org/

Lupus Foundation of America
1300 Piccard Drive, Suite 200, Rockville, MD 20850; (301) 670-9292
http://www.lupus.org/

Lupus Research Institute
149 Madison Avenue, New York NY 10016; (212) 685-4118
http://www.lupusresearchinstitute.org/

The Lupus Site (UK)
http://www.uklupus.co.uk/

MedHelp International
http://www.medhelp.org/HealthTopics/Lupus.html

MedLine (National Library of Medicine)
http://www.nlm.nih.gov/medlineplus/lupus.html
http://www.nlm.nih.gov/medlineplus/ency/article/000435.htm

National Institute of Arthritis and Musculoskeletal and Skin Diseases
http://www.niams.nih.gov/hi/topics/lupus/slehandout
http://www.niams.nih.gov/hi/topics/lupus/shades/index.htm

ProHealth's Lupus Chat
http://www.lupuschat.com/forums/index.cfm?b=Lupus

S.L.E. Foundation
149 Madison Avenue,
New York NY 10016;
(800) 74-LUPUS (745-8787)
http://www.lupusny.org/

Suite 101
http://www.suite101.com/discussions.cfm/4752

University of Missouri
http://www.hsc.missouri.edu/~arthritis/lupus/index.html

University of Washington
http://www.orthop.washington.edu/arthritis/types/lupus/01

OSTEONECROSIS: *SEE* BONES

OSTEOPOROSIS: *SEE* BONES

PAIN MANAGEMENT

American Pain Foundation
Toll-free (888) 615-PAIN
(615-7246)
http://www.painfoundation.org/

American Society of Anesthesiologists
http://www.asahq.org/PatientEducation/managepain.htm

PHYSICIANS AND HOSPITALS
American Board of Medical Specialties
http://www.abms.org/

American Academy of Orthopaedic Surgeons
http://www6.aaos.org/memdir/public/memdir.cfm

American College of Rheumatology
http://www.rheumatology.org/directory/geo.asp

Health Pages
http://www.thehealthpages.com/index.html

Lupus Foundation of America (through local chapters)
http://206.161.82.9/chapters/locator.html

Physician.Info
http://www.physician.info/

State Licensing Boards
http://www.mhsource.com/resource/board.html

US News & World Report
Best Hospitals: Rheumatology
*http://www.usnews.com/usnews/nycu/
health/hosptl/rankings/specihqrheu.htm*

RAYNAUD'S PHENOMENON

**National Institute of
Arthritis, Musculoskeletal, and
Skin Diseases**
*http://www.niams.nih.gov/hi/topics/
raynaud/ar125fs.htm*

RHEUMATIC DISEASES

**American College of
Rheumatology**
1800 Century Place, Atlanta, GA
30345; (404) 633-3777
*http://www.rheumatology.org/public/
factsheets/index.asp?aud=pat*

Arthritis Foundation
http://www.arthritis.org/

Arthritis Society of Canada
http://www.arthritis.ca/

**Centers for Disease Control and
Prevention**
http://www.cdc.gov/nccdphp/arthritis/

Cutting Edge Reports
*http://www.rheuma21st.com/
cutting_index.html*

Hospital for Special Surgery
http://www.rheumatology.hss.edu/

**National Institute of Arthritis and
Musculoskeletal and Skin Diseases**
http://www.niams.nih.gov/

SJÖGREN'S SYNDROME

Dry.Org
http://www.dry.org/

**National Institute of Arthritis and
Musculoskeletal and Skin Diseases**
*http://www.niams.nih.gov/hi/topics/
sjogrens/index.htm*

Sjögren's Syndrome Foundation
8120 Woodmont Avenue,
Bethesda, MD 20814;
(800) 475-6473
http://www.sjogrens.org/

Sjögren's World
http://www.sjsworld.org/

TRAVEL AND HEALTH

**Centers for Disease Control and
Prevention**
- *Health Information for
  International Travel*, a publication
  of the US Government, is
  periodically revised and may
  be ordered from the US
  Government Printing Office
  (GPO): (202) 512-1800 or
  toll-free (866) 512-1800 or
  Web site (*http://www.gpo.gov/*).
- Toll-free, interactive
  International Traveler's
  Information Line (touch-tone
  phone required) provides current
  information on specific
  destinations, including disease
  risks and recommended
  protective measures:
  (877) FYI-TRIP (394–8747)
- *http://www.cdc.gov/travel/*

Index

About the Authors

Sheldon Paul Blau, MD, practices in Long Island, New York. He is clinical professor of medicine at the School of Medicine, State University of New York at Stony Brook and an attending physician at Winthrop University Hospital. A former chief of the division of rheumatic diseases at Nassau County Medical Center (now Nassau University Medical Center), he also chaired the medical center's seminar group in rheumatology. Dr. Blau is a Fellow of the American College of Physicians and a founding Fellow of the American College of Rheumatology.

Dodi Schultz, an award-winning writer, has appeared in many of the major consumer magazines and is author, co-author, or editor of twenty books. She is a past president of the American Society of Journalists and Authors and is a member of the Authors Guild/Authors League of America and the National Association of Science Writers.

Dr. Blau and Ms. Schultz, in addition to the earlier edition of *Living with Lupus*, previously co-authored *Arthritis: Up-to-Date Facts for Patients and Their Families* and *Lupus: The Body Against Itself* (two editions). Dr. Blau is also co-author (with Elaine Fantle Shimberg) of *How to Get Out of the Hospital Alive*, is editor and co-author of the medical text *Emergencies in Rheumatoid Arthritis*, and has published extensively in professional journals. His national television appearances have included *Today* and *Oprah*.